The BIG Book on Bariatric Surgery:
Living Your Best Life After Weight Loss Surgery

Alex Brecher & Natalie Stein

The BIG Book on Bariatric Surgery:
Living Your Best Life After Weight Loss Surgery

Alex Brecher & Natalie Stein

BariatricPal.com

ISBN-13: 978-0-9883882-7-7
Library of Congress Control Number: 2014942874

Introduction

Weight loss surgery is not a single event; it is a lifelong process. Most patients struggle for years with obesity and turn to weight loss surgery only after many unsuccessful diets. For many, the surgery is another chance at life. It does not end when you leave the operating room or when your surgery wounds have healed. It lasts beyond the first year and continues past goal weight. It is a lifelong journey.

Each day leading up to and following weight loss surgery is part of that journey. You focus on protein, measure each bite, chew slowly, and drink plenty of water. You read nutrition labels, go for walks or to the gym, and avoid high-fat, high-sugar foods. You weigh yourself, try on new clothes, and take your vitamin and mineral supplements.

You need a lot of support as a weight loss surgery patient, and you need to know what to expect. Helping patients prepare for and recover from weight loss surgery was the inspiration for our first three books:

- The BIG Book on the Lap-Band: Everything You Need to Know to Lose Weight and Live Well with the Adjustable Gastric Band
- The BIG Book on the Gastric Sleeve: Everything You Need to Know to Lose Weight and Live Well with the Vertical Sleeve Gastrectomy
- The BIG Book on the Gastric Bypass: Everything You Need to Know to Lose Weight and Live Well with the Roux-en-Y Gastric Bypass Surgery

The *BIG Book* trilogy focuses on weight loss surgery itself. The books discuss each weight loss surgery procedure, who should consider it, and how to find a good surgeon. They offer details about recovering from surgery and the post-op diet, dealing with possible complications, and making changes in your life after surgery. The books are mostly for pre-surgery patients and patients who had their surgeries less than a year before.

After we published the *Big Books* on weight loss surgery (WLS), many readers asked us about a book targeted toward WLS veterans. They wanted more about the *how-to* of living after WLS, and little tips that can improve daily life. We listened to readers who needed help making the daily grind a little easier.

This book delivers. It has sections on meal plans, food groups, goal setting, exercise programs, and support systems. It talks about holidays, staying motivated, coping with setbacks and managing challenging family and friends. And, of course, there are recipes.

We asked BariatricPal.com members what they wanted to see in this book, and the most common answer by far was "recipes!" High-protein recipes, dessert recipes, snack recipes, family-friendly recipes, and party recipes. They are all in here, and many of them have easy variations to help you keep your diet interesting. Any reference in **blue** in this book is one that's included in the recipe section at the back of the book.

We sincerely hope you enjoy this book and find it a valuable companion as you lose weight and get healthier.

To your health!

Post-Surgery Diet Progression

Right after surgery, you can consume only liquids. Over the course of several weeks, you progress through different phases before getting to your long-term diet for weight loss and health.

- Clear liquid diet
- Full liquid diet
- Puréed foods diet
- Semi-solid or soft foods diet
- Full solid or regular foods diet

Each stage increases the variety of foods; add only one food at a time, and try only a small amount—you want to be sure that you can tolerate the new food. If the food gives you trouble, try it again in a few weeks. You will eventually be able to tolerate most foods, but some foods, even healthy ones, may continue to cause problems and you will have to avoid them.

Clear Liquid Diet

You will be on a clear liquid diet until 1 to 7 days after surgery, to stay hydrated and to allow your incisions to heal. The diet is nutritionally inadequate, and you should be on it only as long as your surgeon recommends. Sip on fluids and suck ice chips throughout the day.

Figure 1 – Sample meal plan for clear liquid diet

	Sample Day on the Clear Liquid Diet
Breakfast	½ cup sugar-free gelatin
	2 oz. apple juice diluted with 2 oz. water
Snack 1	½ cup sugar-free gelatin
	2 oz. grape juice diluted with 2 oz. water
Lunch	8 oz. (1 cup) mushroom-flavored clear broth
	1 sugar-free ice pop
Snack 2	½ cup Crystal Light
Dinner	½ cup chicken bouillon
	½ cup sugar-free gelatin
	2 oz. grape juice diluted with 2 oz. water
Snack 3	1 sugar-free ice pop
	2 oz. cranberry juice diluted with 2 oz. water

Include	Exclude
✓ Water	X Any solid or semi-solid food
✓ Broth and bouillon	X Nectar
✓ Sugar-free ice pops	X Canned fruit
✓ Sugar-free gelatin	X Milk
✓ Decaffeinated hot tea and unsweetened or diet iced tea	X Protein shakes
✓ Decaffeinated coffee	X Meal replacement beverages
✓ Diluted sports drinks	X Juice with pulp
✓ Pulp-free fruit juices, diluted 1:1 with water (i.e. 4 oz. juice to 1 oz. water)	X Citrus juice and tomato juice (too acidic)
✓ Diet non-carbonated drinks such as Crystal Light and Vitamin Water	X Cream and creamer (e.g. in coffee)
	X Sugar as a sweetener
	X Milk-based coffee drinks such as lattes

Full Liquid Diet

The full liquid diet allows your surgery wounds to continue healing, but it is far more nutritious than the clear liquid diet. Lap-band patients will probably follow this diet from day one after surgery until about a week after surgery. Gastric sleeve and gastric bypass patients are more likely to need the liquid diet for two weeks after surgery. Your surgeon is also likely to ask you to follow the full liquid diet for up to two weeks *before* surgery to jumpstart your weight loss and to prove that you have the motivation and discipline to follow the weight loss surgery diet.

This diet phase is when you start to focus on hitting your 60 to 75 grams of protein per day. Keep sipping on water and other non-caloric fluids to stay hydrated, and limit sugar so that you do not interfere with weight loss or experience dumping syndrome.

Figure 2 – Sample menu full liquid diet

	Sample Day for the Full Liquid Diet
Breakfast	8 oz. low-fat milk and 1 scoop sugar-free protein powder
Snack 1	8 oz. sugar-free protein shake
Lunch	12 oz. low-fat milk with 10 grams sugar-free chocolate-flavored protein powder
Snack 2	½ cup sugar-free pudding 1 ice pop
Dinner	8 oz. (1 cup) strained cream of mushroom soup made with milk and protein powder
Snack 3	Hot cocoa with protein powder

Include	Exclude
✓ Everything on the clear liquid diet	X Bread, pasta, rice
✓ 1% low-fat or skim milk	X Nuts, beans, seeds
✓ Skim milk powder	X Meats, poultry, fish
✓ Unsweetened soymilk and almond milk	X Cheese
✓ Protein shakes and powders (see BP Book Protein for guidelines)	X Fruit and vegetables
✓ Sugar-free hot cocoa	X Ice cream and frozen yogurt
✓ Strained cream soups	X Sugar, honey and syrups
✓ Sugar-free pudding	X Cream of wheat, cream of rice, oatmeal (ask your surgeon)
	X Applesauce

Puréed Foods Diet

You can gradually add puréed and very smooth foods back into your diet. Lap-band patients may complete this phase as soon as two weeks after surgery, while vertical sleeve gastrectomy and gastric bypass patients are more likely to need up to four weeks before moving on to Phase 4. Each meal or snack should be 1 to 2 oz. for gastric bypass patients. VSG and lap-band patients may be able to eat 6 oz., but you should not stuff your sleeve or pouch. At this time, the food groups in your menus should be approaching the daily goals for your long-term high-protein weight loss surgery diet.

The puréed foods phase lets you practice the healthy behaviors that should become habits. Eat slowly, chew thoroughly, and eat your protein first at each meal. Also, choose nutritious foods, and do not drink fluids within 30 minutes of eating food. To reduce side effects, add in only one new food at a time.

Include
- ✓ Liquids allowed during Stages 1 and 2
- ✓ Puréed fat-free cottage cheese
- ✓ Fat-free plain or no-sugar-added yogurt
- ✓ Silken tofu
- ✓ Puréed cream and thin soups
- ✓ Puréed watery potatoes and sweet potatoes (no strings)
- ✓ Eggs and liquid egg substitutes
- ✓ Ripe mashed bananas
- ✓ Canned pears and peaches
- ✓ Unsweetened applesauce
- ✓ Well-cooked non-fibrous vegetables
- ✓ Puréed oatmeal, Cream of Wheat, and Malt-O-Meal
- ✓ Baby food meat

Exclude
- X Tough or stringy meat
- X Bread and cold cereal
- X Most grains, such as rice and pasta
- X Nuts and seeds, peanut and nut butter
- X Vegetables/fruit with seeds or peel
- X Fruit jam
- X High-calorie unhealthy choices, e.g. ice cream and butter
- X Crackers, pretzels, and popcorn
- X Raw vegetables and fruit
- X Potentially sticky foods, e.g. pasta and rice

Figure 3 – Sample days on puréed foods diet

The serving sizes shown may be larger than what you need. P=Protein D=Dairy V=Vegetable F=Fruit S=Starch Ft=Fat

	Day 1 Sample	Day 2 Sample
Breakfast	½ cup oatmeal made with fat-free milk and 1 scoop protein powder ½ cup plain Greek yogurt	¼ cup fat-free ricotta cheese ½ cup puréed canned pears
Snack 1	¼ cup cooked liquid eggs or 2 egg whites	8 oz. low-carb protein shake
Lunch	½ cup puréed vegetable soup with 1 scoop unflavored protein powder ½ cup puréed winter squash with 1 tsp. margarine	½ cup soft tofu ½ cup puréed canned or well-cooked carrots
Dinner	½ cup puréed zucchini ½ cup baby food chicken with gravy	½ cup mashed potatoes made with fat-free milk and 1 tsp. olive oil ½ cup fat-free cottage cheese
Snack 2	½ cup plain Greek yogurt ½ cup stewed peeled apples with cinnamon and calorie-free sweetener, with 1 scoop protein powder	½ cup cream of wheat made with skim milk and extra protein powder or powdered skim milk
Totals	5 P, 2 D, 3 V, 1 F, 1 S, 1 Ft	5 P, 2 D, 2 V, 1 F, 1 S, 1 Ft

Semi-Soft or Solid Foods Diet

This phase lets you continue adding foods gradually back into your diet. The phase may be as short as a week for most patients. In this phase, try to reduce the liquid calories that you take in if you are still depending on protein shakes. Instead, try to get your protein from food sources. Also, move away from pureéeing your foods, because puréed foods are less satisfying than foods with texture. Avoid sharp, tough, fibrous and sticky foods, and cook meat thoroughly.

Figure 4 – Foods on the semi-solid or soft foods diet

Include

- ✓ Foods allowed on the puréed foods diet
- ✓ Ripe fruit without peel or seeds
- ✓ Canned tuna and salmon
- ✓ Lean ground turkey, chicken and beef
- ✓ Crab meat
- ✓ Baked fish (beware of bones)
- ✓ Lean deli meat
- ✓ Well-cooked beans and lentils
- ✓ Canned chicken
- ✓ Reduced-fat cheese
- ✓ Well-cooked pasta and rice
- ✓ Nut butters and peanut butter (lap-band patients may need to avoid)

Exclude

- X Tough or stringy meat
- X Hard foods such as crackers, pretzels, cold cereal, rice cakes, chips and popcorn
- X Nuts, seeds, and peanuts
- X Raw vegetables
- X Fibrous/stringy vegetables such as asparagus
- X Potentially sticky foods such as pasta and rice
- X Meat, poultry, or fish with bones, skin, or gristle
- X Bread

Figure 5 – Sample menus on the semi-solid foods diet

	Day 1 Sample	Day 2 Sample
Breakfast	2 egg whites scrambled with skim milk and 1 tsp. margarine 1 oz. fat-free cheese ½ cup cantaloupe	1 packet instant oatmeal made with skim milk and added non-fat milk powder ½ cup canned pears
Snack 1	2 oz. extra lean turkey breast	2 hard-boiled egg whites
Lunch	½ cup cottage cheese ½ cup cooked peas	2 oz. imitation crab meat ½ cup cooked carrots
Dinner	2 oz. lean ground turkey ½ small boiled sweet potato, peeled ½ cup canned green beans	2 oz. canned chicken ¼ cup white rice, well-cooked ½ cup well-cooked frozen cauliflower florets with 1 tsp. margarine
Snack 2	¼ cup fat-free ricotta cheese ½ cup cooked beets	3 oz. light silken tofu blended with ½ cup frozen peaches
Totals	4 P, 3 D, 3 V, 1 S, 1 F	5 P, 1 D, 2 V, 2 F, 2 S, 1 Ft

Transitioning to the Regular Diet

The liquid, puréed foods, and semi-solid diets let your surgery wounds heal and lay the foundation for better weight loss later. These are a few reminders for this period:

- ✓ Eat only the foods that your surgeon allows in each phase.
- ✓ If a food does not agree with you, try it again in a week or two.
- ✓ Emphasize protein at each meal and snack.
- ✓ After the liquid diet, limit or eliminate caloric beverages.

Lap-band patients may start the solid foods diet as soon as three weeks after surgery, and gastric bypass and vertical sleeve gastrectomy patients may start eating solid foods within four weeks of surgery. However, each patient heals at a different rate. Take as long as you need to get through the liquid, puréed food, or semi-solid food stages before you start on solid foods.

The solid foods diet is your long-term weight loss surgery diet. These tips can help you lose more weight and stay better nourished with this diet.

- ✓ Make progress gradually. Add in only one new food at a time, and start with a single bite.
- ✓ When you start adding solid foods, start with low-fiber options.
- ✓ Gradually increase your emphasis on high-protein, high-fiber, high-nutrient foods.
- ✓ Practice eating slowly.

Basic Diet Rules for Weight Loss

Following your WLS diet lets you lose weight and keep it off. These are the basic dietary guidelines for long-term weight control and health after bariatric surgery.

- ☐ Eat slowly to aid weight loss and prevent complications. See tips below.
- ☐ Chew thoroughly before swallowing.
- ☐ Eat protein first. Follow with vegetables, fruit, and then starches.
- ☐ Avoid fluids within 30 minutes before or after meals.
- ☐ Drink at least 64 oz. (eight 8-oz. cups) of water or other low-calorie fluids per day.
- ☐ Make low-calorie nutritious food choices.
- ☐ Do not overeat. Portion sizes are much smaller after surgery than they were before. They might be just a few ounces after surgery, or as much as a cup with the lap-band when you are a ways out from surgery.
- ☐ Introduce new foods slowly. Take one bite and try only one new food at a time.
- ☐ Eat at the table. Eat only your 3 to 6 meals and snacks, with no "grazing" in between.
- ☐ Eat "mindfully." Enjoy your food and the eating environment, such as your company and the atmosphere. Ignore distractions, such as work or TV or internet.
- ☐ Vary your diet to prevent boredom and add more nutrients.

Choose nutritious foods instead of junk foods

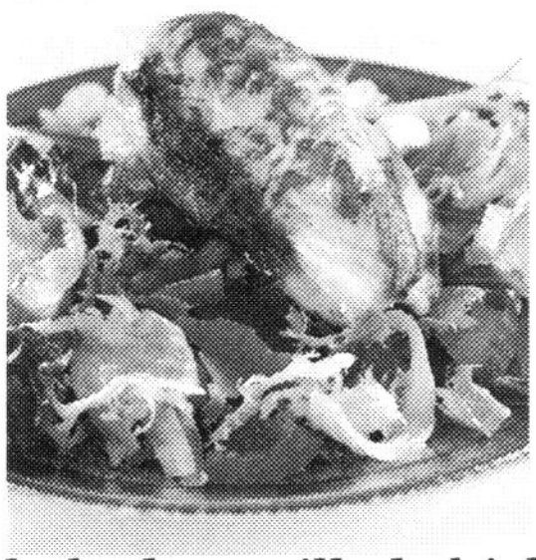

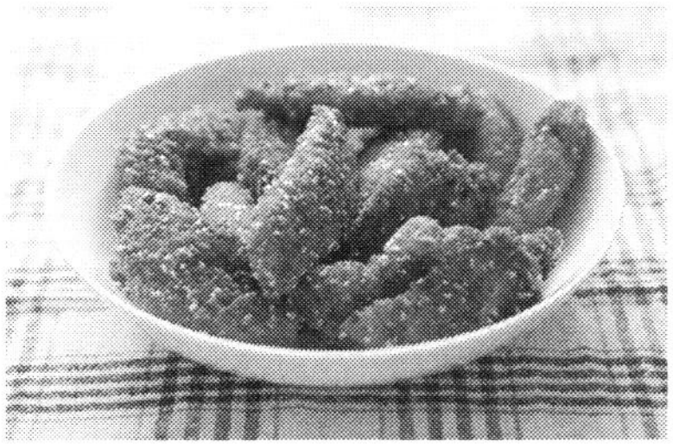

Choose baked or grilled chicken breast instead of chicken strips—it's higher in protein and lower in fat, carbohydrates, and calories.

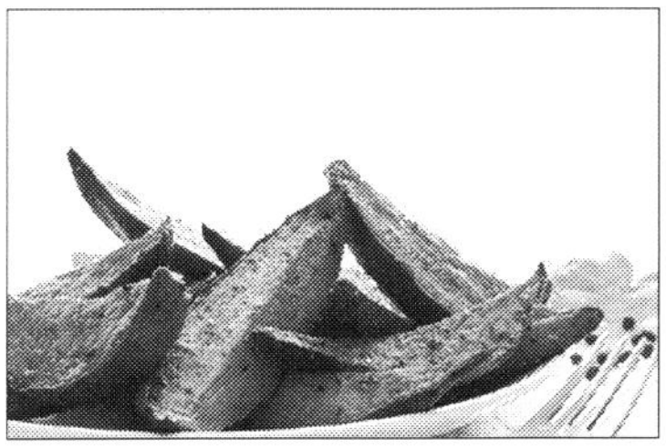

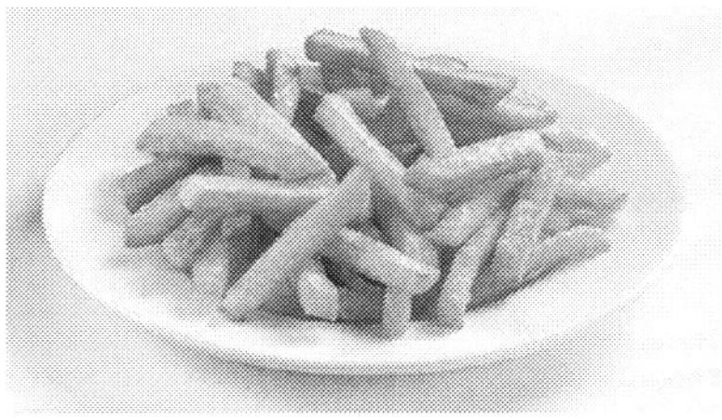

Enjoy a baked, grilled, or roasted sweet potato or yam instead of French fries—you'll consume about one-third the calories and far less sodium and fat. Choose grilled chicken breast instead of

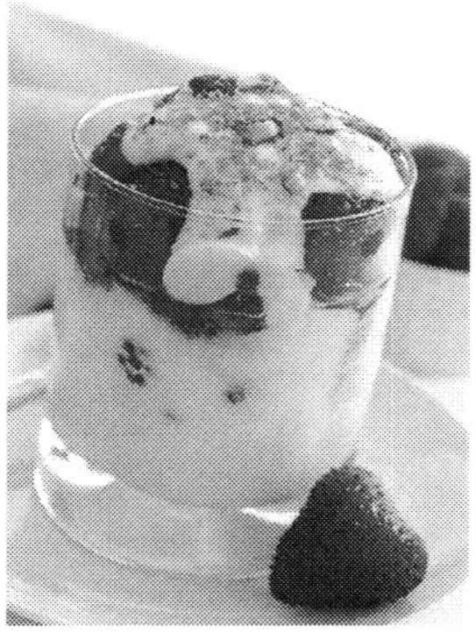

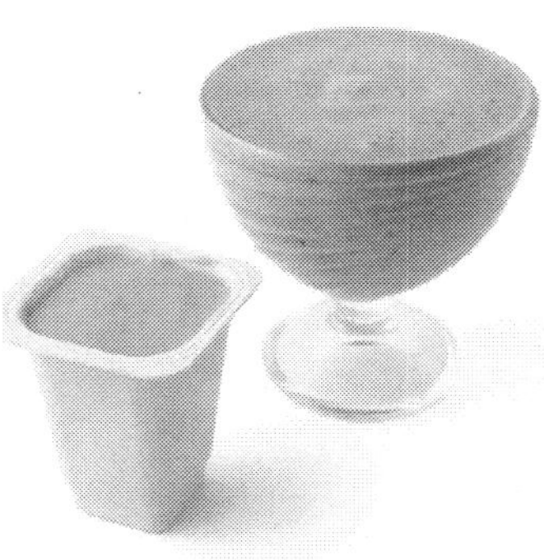

Choose non-fat plain Greek yogurt with fresh fruit instead of fruit-flavored low-fat yogurt—it has more protein and fiber and fewer calories and sugar.

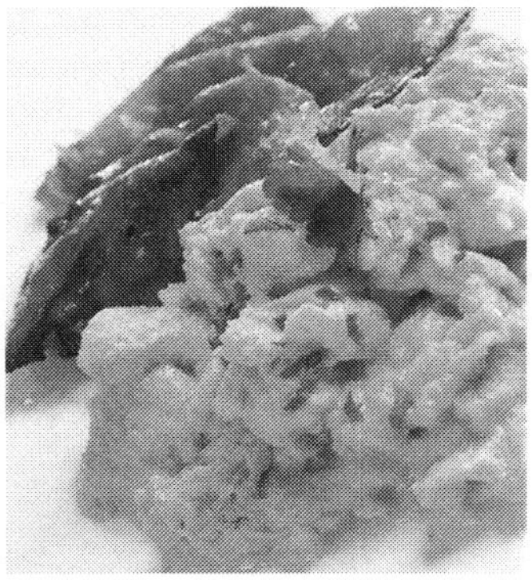

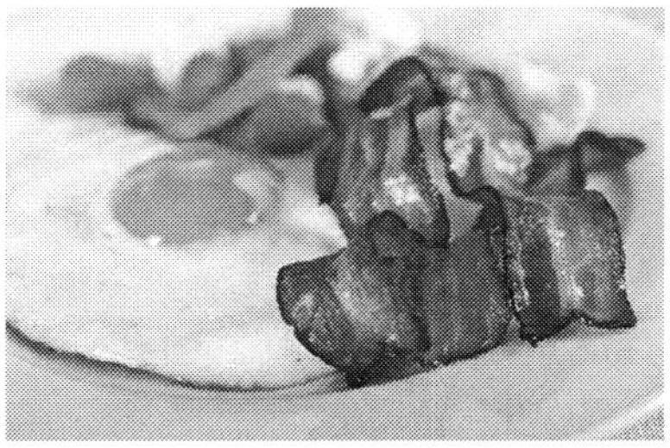

Choose scrambled eggs or egg whites and lean ham cooked with olive oil instead of whole eggs cooked in butter and served with bacon—it's lower in calories and in saturated fat.

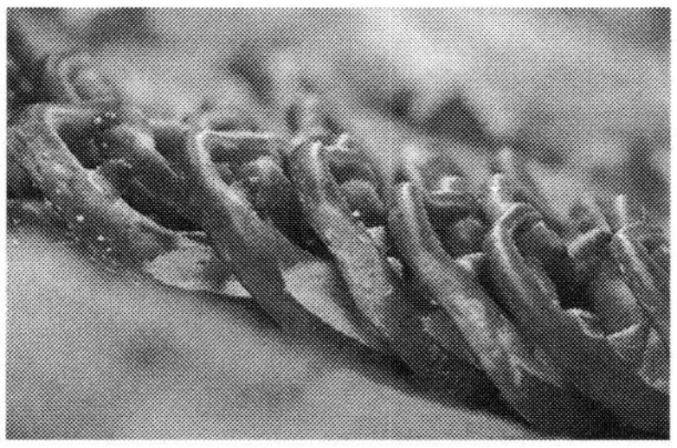

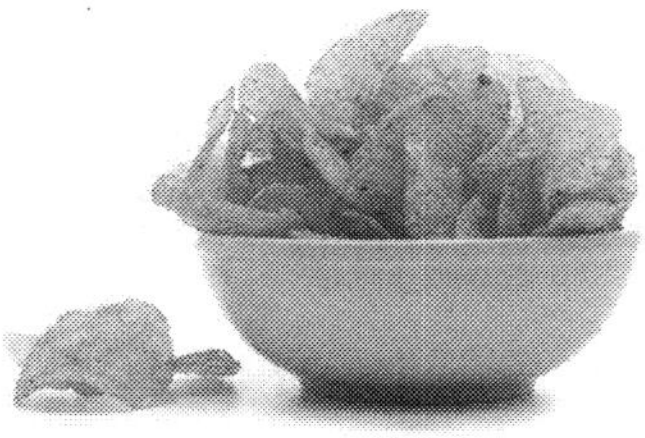

Choose whole grain pretzels over potato chips—you'll save on both calories and fat.

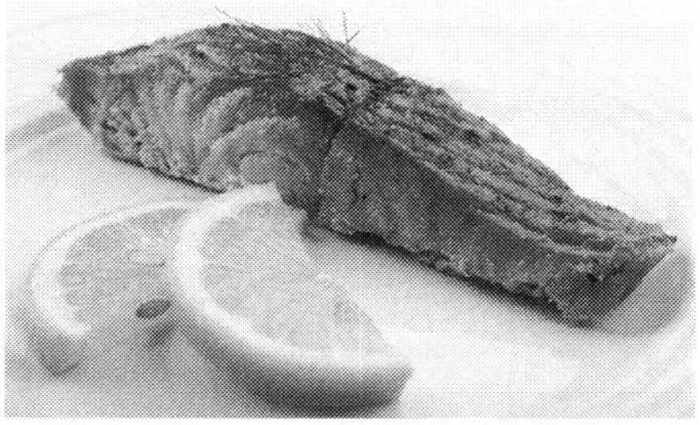

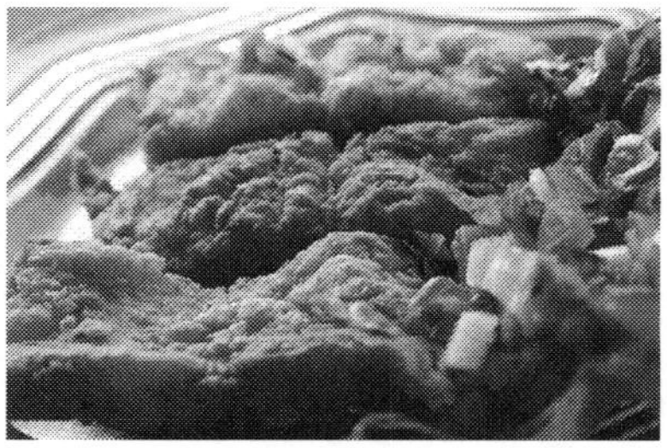

Enjoy a serving of seared herb-crusted albacore or grilled salmon with dill instead of having crab cakes or fried fish with coleslaw—salmon and albacore are higher in protein, fiber, and hearth-healthy omega-3 fats, and much lower in calories and total fat.

Tips for Eating Slowly

You need to eat more slowly after surgery than you did before. Eating too fast can stall weight loss, both by causing you to overeat and also by stretching your small stomach pouch or sleeve. Fast eating can also cause complications such as nausea, dumping syndrome in gastric bypass patients and, in sleeve patients, early satiety or uncomfortable feelings of fullness after you have not eaten very much. Practice these strategies to eat more slowly.

- Make each meal last at least 20 to 30 minutes without going back for seconds. That is how long it takes for your brain to recognize that you are full. Set a timer or watch the clock to make sure you give your stomach a chance to tell your brain that you are full.
- Count your chews. Chew each bite 30 times before swallowing. This is tedious, but it will help you get into the habit of chewing until food is mushy.
- Take small bites. Children's utensils such as a shallow spoon and small fork can help.
- Eat slower than the others at your table.

Other Guidelines for a Healthy WLS Lifestyle

- Take your multivitamin and other supplements each day.
- Exercise according to your doctor's recommendations.
- Plan and log your meals. (see BP Book Plan your Meals)
- Set realistic weight loss and other goals (See BP Book Head Games). Work toward them, but remember to savor the journey.
- Keep attending your support group meetings and frequently re-evaluate your support system to make sure it still meets your needs (See BP Book Plateau Regain)
- Be honest with yourself in all areas, including diet, exercise, your feelings, and your physical and emotional needs.
- Ask for help when you need it.

Special Guidelines for Lap-Band Patients

- Eat three meals per day, with snacks only if your surgeon or dietitian recommends it.
- Monitor your hunger and comfort to make sure you stay in the "green zone" (see BP Book Green Zone).
- Be ready to spend a day or two on a liquid or puréed foods diet after a fill.

The adjustable gastric band is the least invasive procedure, and it does not interfere with nutrient absorption. However, lap-band patients can have many long-term dietary restrictions. Sticky and gummy or chewy foods can block the narrow opening between your stoma and your larger stomach pouch below. Gristly and stringy foods can get caught in the band. Approach suspect foods cautiously or avoid them altogether, and be sure to chew them thoroughly before swallowing.

Figure 6 – Troublesome foods for lap-band patients

Sticky or Chewy: Raisins Other dried fruit Candy Fried foods	**Gristly or Sharp:** Dry meat, poultry, or fish Tough meat such as steak and pork chops Sausage Shrimp Nuts and peanuts Seeds
Gummy or Doughy: Pasta Rice Bread Other starchy foods Hot dogs	**Stringy or Fibrous:** Celery Other raw vegetables Salad Citrus fruits Fresh pineapple Corn Broccoli Asparagus

The band works by slowing the passage of food from your stoma (the small portion of your stomach pouch above the band) to the rest of your stomach. Liquids pass right through the band and do not keep you as full as solid foods. You should avoid caloric fluids and semi-liquid calorie sources. This is true even of nutritious semi-liquids such as soup, unless you are having trouble tolerating solid foods and are on a liquid or puréed food diet. As long as you are tolerating solid foods on your usual lap-band diet, you should still avoid or limit:

- Fluids with calories (See BP Book Fluids)
- Soup, unless you are drinking broth or bouillon to meet your fluid needs between meals
- Ice cream
- Salad dressing
- Thin yogurt
- Applesauce

Special Guidelines for Vertical Sleeve Gastrectomy Patients

Early satiety is a greater threat to sleeve patients because of the small size of your sleeve. Early satiety can strike at any time, making you feel uncomfortably full after eating only one or two bites. When it happens, your meal is over. Vertical sleeve gastrectomy patients:

- Should eat five or six small meals per day.
- May need protein supplements in the form of powders or even shakes.
- Should make high-nutrient foods a high priority.

Because of their sharp edges, crunchy foods may irritate the line where your sleeve is fastened shut. You may need to avoid nuts, seeds, and chips (tortilla, corn, and potato). These foods may be okay a few months after surgery, but one or more of them may be troublesome for longer (or forever). Introduce only a single bite at a time, and chew it well. If a certain food is troublesome, try it again in a few weeks if your doctor approves. By that time, it may be tolerable.

Special Guidelines for Roux-en-Y Gastric Bypass Patients

Roux-en-Y gastric bypass patients have a higher risk of dumping syndrome. To prevent dumping syndrome:

- Avoid high-sugar foods. Stick to foods with no more than 5 grams of sugar per serving.
- Avoid high-fat foods including fried foods, fatty cold cuts, full-fat cheeses, and pastries.
- Eat slowly and do not overeat.

Avoid stretching your pouch to promote better long-term success after RYGB.

- Eat four to six high-protein mini-meals daily, or three meals and one to three snacks.
- Keep portions small.
- Stop eating when you are full.

□

Meal and Menu Planning

Menus

Meal planning is one of the most important things you can do after weight loss surgery, but it can be challenging at the beginning. After planning daily or weekly menus for a while, you might find yourself in a rut. These are some considerations for your meal plans.

- ☐ Each day's menus should provide enough protein and other nutrients.
- ☐ Menus should be low-calorie, low-sugar, and low-fat so you can lose weight.
- ☐ Menus should vary and include a wide range of foods so you get a range of nutrients and do not get bored.
- ☐ You should plan three meals per day, plus up to three snacks if your nutritionist suggests them. Lap-band patients are more likely to have only three meals, while gastric sleeve patients are more likely to need six small meals or snacks per day. Gastric bypass patients fall in between.

The following daily goals will get you close to 1,200 to 1,400 calories and 60 to 70 grams of protein. Your surgeon or nutritionist may have slightly different recommendations.

- Protein (P) 5 to 6 servings
- Dairy (D) 2 to 3 servings
- Vegetables (V) 2 to 4 servings
- Fruit (F) 2 servings
- Starch (S) 2 to 5 servings
- Fat (Ft) 2 to 3 servings

You can divide these up in many ways, but be sure to include protein at most meals and snacks, especially breakfast. The list below shows two different daily meal patterns and some foods that you could eat for each one.

Meal pattern 1 has three meals and one snack.

- ☐ Breakfast: 2 P, 1 F
- ☐ Lunch: 2 P, 1 S, 1 Ft, 1 V
- ☐ Dinner: 2 P, 1 D, 1 V, 1 F
- ☐ Snack: 1 D, 1 S

Meal pattern 2 has three meals and three snacks.

- ☐ Breakfast: 1 P, 1 D, 1 F
- ☐ Snack 1: 1 P, 1 V, 1 Ft
- ☐ Lunch: 1 P, 1 V, 1 S, 1 Ft
- ☐ Snack 2: 1 P, 1 Ft
- ☐ Dinner: 1 P, 2 V, 1 F, 1 Ft
- ☐ Snack 3: 1 P, 1 S

Figure 7 – Sample meal patterns and possible menus

	Meal Pattern 1	Sample Day Based on the Pattern
Breakfast	2 protein 1 fruit	1 low-fat turkey breakfast sausage 2 scrambled egg whites 1 cup strawberries
Lunch	1 vegetable 2 protein 1 starch 1 fat	2 cups mixed greens 2 hard-boiled egg whites and 2 oz. lean turkey, chopped in salad ½ small low-carb or low-calorie bagel 2 tbsp. reduced-fat dressing
Dinner	2 protein 1 dairy 1 vegetable 1 fat 1 fruit	1 serving of **canned salmon bake** made with pecan crust 1 cup watermelon
Snack	1 dairy 1 starch	1 packet plain instant oatmeal made with fat-free milk

	Meal Pattern 2	Sample Day Based on the Patten
Breakfast	1 protein 1 dairy 1 fruit	1 small veggie burger or 2 oz. lean ground turkey 1 oz. fat-free cheese ½ grapefruit
Snack 1	1 protein 1 veggie 1 fat	Egg, ranch dressing, raw veggies (or cooked broccoli or green beans if you can't eat raw veggies)
Lunch	1 vegetable 1 starch 1 protein 1 fat	1 cup sprouts and/or shredded lettuce ½ whole-grain pita 2 oz. lean turkey breast 1 tbsp. reduced-fat cream cheese
Snack 2	1 protein 1 fat	**Tuna salad** with low-fat mayo
Dinner	1 protein 2 vegetables 1 starch 1 fat	½ cup black beans 1 cup shredded lettuce ½ cup canned stewed tomatoes ½ cup cooked brown rice 2 tbsp. guacamole
Snack 3	1 protein 1 starch	¼ cup fat-free ricotta cheese ½ whole-grain English muffin

Figure 8 shows a full week of sample meal plans with three meals and two snacks per day. You can adjust the snacks to meet your needs. For example, lap-band patients who eat only three meals per day might make their meals a little bigger and skip the snacks. Gastric sleeve patients may need an extra snack, but might keep the meals a little smaller. Your individual needs may be slightly different, so talk to a nutritionist about recommended adjustments to portion sizes.

Figure 8 – Sample 7-day menu with three meals and two snacks

Day 1	Day 2	Day 3	Day 4	Day 5	Day 6	Day 7
1 serving non-fat Greek plain yogurt 1 cup blueberries ½ cup Fiber One	1 slice high-fiber low-calorie toast 1 tsp. margarine ½ cup fat-free cottage cheese	2 scrambled egg whites (or ¼ cup egg substitute), cooking spray 1 cup mushrooms 1 oz. shredded low-fat cheese	1 lean turkey or meatless breakfast patty 2 cooked egg whites 1 orange	½ cup silken tofu scrambled with 1 cup tomatoes, onions, and peppers and 1 tsp. olive oil	2 egg whites scrambled with 2 oz. lean ham 1 cup spinach	packet plain instant oatmeal 1 scoop protein powder ½ sliced banana
hard-boiled egg whites	1 cup carrot sticks 1 tbsp. peanut butter	1 pear 1 oz. pecans	1 serving **tuna salad**	2 oz. turkey breast 1 slice low-calorie bread 1 tbsp. avocado	½ banana 1 tbsp. peanut butter	1 low-fat cheese stick 1 cup carrot sticks
2 oz. deli ham rolled up with 1 oz. fat-free cheese 1 cup kale chips	½ cup **bean salad** 2 oz. salmon 1 cup celery sticks	Salad with 2 cups raw spinach leaves 1 tbsp. light balsamic vinaigrette 2 oz. grilled chicken breast ½ cup artichoke hearts	small l high-fiber wrap or tortilla ½ cup fat-free low-sodium canned refried beans 2 small slices avocado 2 tbsp. salsa	½ cup fat-free cottage cheese 1 oz. almonds 1 cup cantaloupe	1 serving red pepper **Greek yogurt dip** 1 cup cucumber slices 1 oz. whole-grain crackers	2 cups mixed greens 2 oz. tuna 1 cup diced tomatoes 2 tbsp. Greek yogurt dressing
1 small apple 1 tbsp. peanut butter	1 small pear 1 oz. low-fat cheese	1 container plain non-fat Greek yogurt	¼ cup fat-free ricotta cheese ½ banana	6 medium shrimp 1 cup cherry tomatoes	½ cup winter squash	½ oz. nuts ½ cup fat-free cottage cheese
2 oz. ground turkey breast 1 low-calorie hamburger bun 1 cup grilled vegetables (about ½ small eggplant or 1 small zucchini, 1 tbsp. mustard	1 cup **chicken stir fry** ½ cup well-cooked brown rice 1 cup grapes	2 oz. grilled tilapia ⅓ cup whole-wheat couscous 1 cup berries	1 serving "fried chicken" Recipe page XX ½ cup smashed cauliflower (Recipe page XXX) ½ cup cooked greens	2 oz. extra lean steak ½ sweet potato ½ cup steamed green beans	2 oz. grilled chicken breast 1 small grilled zucchini with 1 tsp. olive oil 1 cup watermelon	½ cup whole wheat pasta 2 oz. extra lean ground turkey ½ cup tomato sauce ½ cup steamed broccoli
5 P, 2 D, 2 V, 2 F, 2 S, 1 F	4 P, 2 D, 3 V, 2 F, 2 S, 2 Ft	4 P, 2 D, 3 V, 2 F, 2 S, 1 Ft	5 P, 1 D, 2 V, 2 F, 2 S, 2 Ft	5 P, 1 D, 2 V, 2 F, 2 S, 2 Ft	5 P, 2 D, 3 V, 2 S, 1 F, 2 Ft	4 P, 2 D, 5 V, 1 F, 2 S, 1 Ft

You can also plan menus by mixing and matching healthy meals; the following table shows some high-protein options. Choose a breakfast, lunch, and dinner. To satisfy your hunger, get more nutrients and hit your food group goals, add one or two servings of vegetables, fruit, or healthy starches. You may also need one or more high-protein snacks.

Figure 9 – High-protein low-calorie breakfast, lunch, and dinner ideas

Breakfast	Lunch	Dinner
High protein French toast	Spinach, egg and cheese crepe	Grilled chicken or shrimp skewers
Protein powder pancakes	Chunky low-fat chili	Turkey stuffed portabella mushrooms
Breakfast sandwich on English muffin	English muffin pizza	Meatloaf
Oatmeal breakfast bar	Chicken breast with hummus on ½ whole-grain pita	Spaghetti squash with tomato sauce and meatballs
High-fiber cereal and yogurt	Chicken quesadilla on low-carb tortilla with low-fat cheese	Macaroni and cheese
Fat-free cream cheese and smoked salmon on ½ whole-wheat bagel	Whole wheat pretzels with peanut butter	Zucchini pancakes
Cottage cheese pancakes	Southwestern lettuce wraps with lean ground turkey, salsa, and tomatoes	Family taco bar (everyone can serve themselves their favorite toppings)

You can always keep it simple. Use the food lists at the end of this book to help you assemble a balanced meal or snack with no cooking required. Just choose one or two servings of protein or dairy foods and add one or two servings of vegetables, fruit or starches, and you're ready to eat.

Make Your Meal Plan!

Print a couple of copies of the blank meal plan from the next page. Use it to plan nutritious low-calorie meals and help you make your weekly grocery list.

	Breakfast	Snack 1	Lunch	Snack 2	Dinner	Totals
Day 1						
Day 2						
Day 3						
Day 4						
Day 5						
Day 6						
Day 7						

Timing Your Meals

Careful timing is important when you are scrambling to get your three to six meals, 64 oz. fluid, and dietary supplements each day. This following schedule shows how to space your meals and snacks, keep your liquids separate from your fluids, and maximize absorption of nutritional supplements.

- ☐ 6:30 a.m. 1 cup water
- ☐ 7:00 a.m. breakfast with multivitamin with calcium
- ☐ 8:30 a.m. 1 cup water
- ☐ 9:30 a.m. 1 cup water with iron and vitamin B-12 supplement
- ☐ 10:00 a.m. snack #1
- ☐ 11:00 a.m. 1 cup water
- ☐ Noon: lunch with a multivitamin with calcium (if your doctor has recommended that you take two daily multivitamins)
- ☐ 1:00 p.m. 1 cup water
- ☐ 2:00 p.m. 1 cup water
- ☐ 3:00 p.m. snack #2
- ☐ 4:30 p.m. 1 cup water
- ☐ 6:00 p.m. dinner with a calcium supplement
- ☐ 7:00 p.m. 1 cup water

Planning and Logging Your Weight Loss Surgery Diet

From before surgery through long-term maintenance of goal weight, you are far more likely to have better results if you plan your meals and snacks in advance and you log what you actually ate. Planning and logging help you:

- Meet your requirements for protein and other nutrients.
- Stick to the low-calorie foods that are part of your weight loss surgery diet.
- Prevent last-minute decisions to eat unhealthy foods.
- Always have enough weight loss surgery diet foods on hand.
- Exercise regularly.

You can plan by:

- Organizing your menus and scheduling workouts.
- Making the most of your grocery trips.
- Preparing food ahead of time.
- Planning for the unexpected.
- Making food logging a habit.

Planning Your Menus and Workouts

You can write down the next day's menu each night, or take some time each week to create your weekly menus. BP Book Meal Planning has menu templates, sample daily menus, and guidelines for creating your own nutritious menus. Your daily or weekly menu planning session is also a good time to create your exercise schedule for the next day or week.

Effective Grocery Shopping

After weight loss surgery, you are probably doing most of your own food preparation rather than depending on fast food, take-out, and restaurant dining. These tips can help you ensure that your efforts translate into the weight loss results you deserve!

- Use a shopping list. If you do weekly meal planning, the time when you plan your menus is a good time to make your list. Another option is to keep a running list on a pad of paper in the kitchen or a white board on the refrigerator so you can add items to the list as you think of them.
- If you go grocery shopping only once a week, be sure you get enough fruits and vegetables. If you can't get enough fresh produce to get through the week, you can stock up on frozen fruits and vegetables. Another option is to go to a farmers' market or even back to the grocery store mid-way through the week to re-stock your supply. Fresh chicken, meat, and fish can be frozen and thawed as you need them.
- Buy foods that make sticking to your weight loss surgery diet easier by saving time. Pre-grilled chicken breast strips, pre-shaped ground turkey burger patties, marinated cuts of meat or poultry, liquid egg whites, pre-cut ready-to-cook vegetables, baby carrots and bagged salads are a few examples.

Preparing Food Ahead of Time

Preparing food ahead of time helps you stick to your healthy eating plan even on busy days. Besides buying easy-to-prepare foods, you can also save time by preparing some foods ahead of time. Once a week, dedicate some time to preparing for the upcoming week.

- Make entire recipes and freeze them in single-serving portions to defrost when you need them. You can do this with almost any dish, including pastas, sauces, soups, and stews. Try bariatric-friendly **chili** and cooked vegetables, such as high-protein puréed or **smashed cauliflower**.
- Cook chicken breast, pork tenderloin, beef round or fish, cut it into small portions of 1 to 3 oz. and freeze.
- Hard-boil a dozen or more eggs and keep them in the fridge.
- Wash, peel and cut fresh vegetables to snack on or use in recipes. They will stay good in the refrigerator for a couple of days.
- Weigh, measure or count out portions of foods to eat later. Examples include placing 1-oz. servings of breakfast cereal or low-fat cheese in baggies or containers, freezing small baggies or containers of ¾-cup servings of frozen blueberries and putting 1-tbsp. portions of peanut butter in small containers to take for lunches. You can also count your foods, such as 6-nut portions of almonds, in advance.

Plan for the Unforeseeable

You cannot plan for unpredictable events, but you can prevent them from throwing you off your weight loss surgery diet. Keep healthy foods on hand so that you can always be sure to have something healthy to eat regardless of the situation.

- Keep healthy foods at home, in case you do not make the grocery store as planned.
- At work, in case you leave home before breakfast, work through lunch, face tempting refreshments in meetings or at the front desk, or stay at work later than expected.
- In the car, in case you are stuck in traffic, go to the gym, or make a detour.

The first priority is to have enough protein on hand. Complete your meal or snack with other healthy options, such as vegetables, grains, and fruits. Following are some non-perishable items that can be stored at room temperature. If you are stocking up for work or home, frozen and refrigerated foods can also come to your rescue at the last minute.

Non-perishable protein ideas:

- Canned or pouch tuna, salmon, chicken, or sardines
- Canned beans, such as garbanzo, kidney, black or fat-free refried
- Roasted soybeans (soynuts)
- Protein bars
- Shelf-stable (boxed) silken tofu
- Protein powder

Non-perishable vegetables, grains, fruits, and nuts:

- Low-sodium, no-sugar-added canned vegetables such as green beans, carrots, peas, and tomatoes

- ☐ Whole-grain cereal
- ☐ Peanut butter (except lap-band patients if you cannot tolerate it)
- ☐ Instant oatmeal packets that you can make with hot water and protein powder
- ☐ Canned fruit in water or its own juice (no sugar added)
- ☐ Unsweetened applesauce that you can eat with protein powder mixed in
- ☐ Peanuts, mixed nuts, or trail mix (lap-band patients: be cautious)
- ☐ Microwave popcorn (100-calorie packs or low-fat options); lap-band patients, be cautious)
- ☐ Whole-grain pretzels, crackers, pita chips, or rice cakes

Don't forget to store a can opener with your canned goods!

Making Food Logging a Habit

Food logging, also known as journaling or tracking, is another habit that increases your chances of success after weight loss surgery. The habit of journaling:

- ☐ Keeps you accountable
- ☐ Lets you see how well your actual dietary intake compares with your planned menu and your recommendations
- ☐ Helps you identify patterns, such as the situations that lead you to eat poorly or which foods may trigger side effects, such as dumping syndrome or GERD

A traditional food journal is on paper. See below for a sample journal excerpt. Paper food diaries are easy to fill out, but they do not calculate your nutrient intake for you. Below is an example of a simple food journal excerpt, with a sample meal.

Figure 10 – Sample food journal

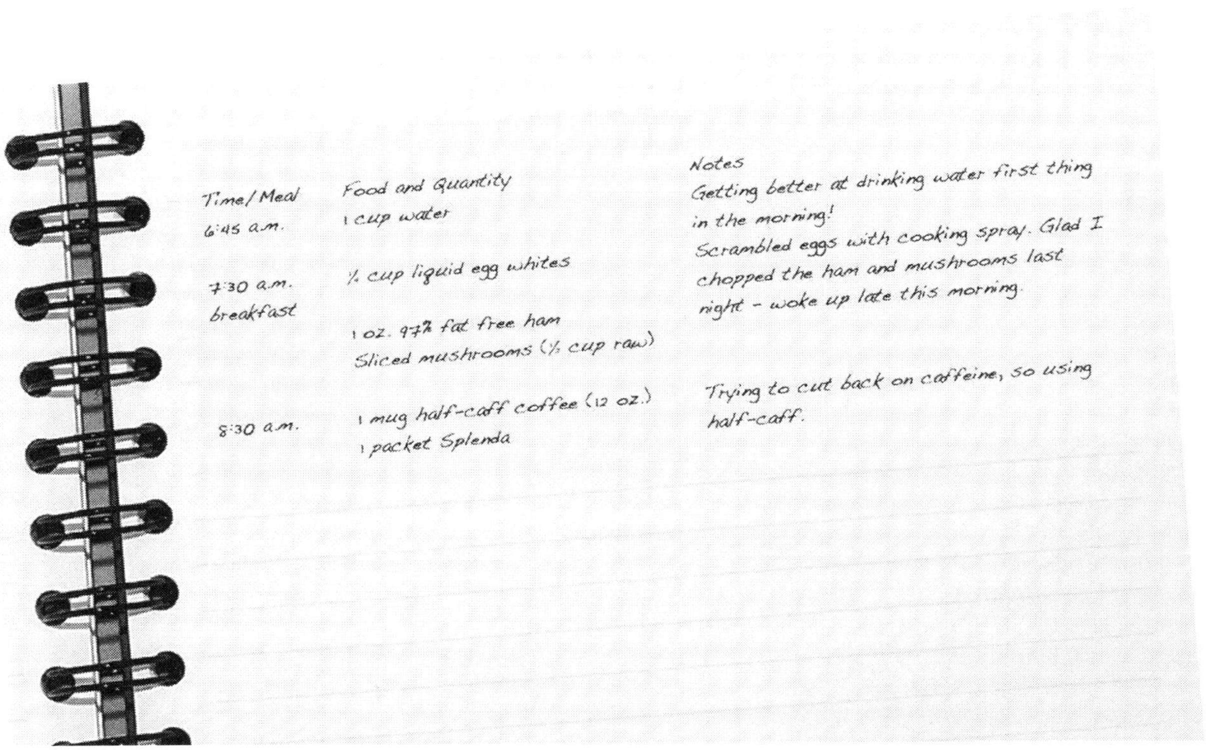

Many online food tracking programs have these advantages:

- Calculate calories, nutrients, and food groups for you.
- Provide reports such as your protein intake over the past week, or how your intake compares with your goals.
- Link to other personal data such as weight and body measurements, a blog, exercise activities and calories, and a personal profile.
- Are within communities where other members make their journals public, so you can get ideas from other weight loss surgery patients.
- Offer the option of publicly sharing your food journal so other community members can comment on it and provide suggestions.

Complete your food journal at least once a day, preferably after each meal and snack. This reduces your chances of forgetting foods and helps keep you motivated. Online food logs make frequent logging easier, because you can access them from your smartphone or any device with internet access.

The information that online trackers provides can be overwhelming. Do not try to monitor everything; just pick out a few of the more important numbers to watch. These may include:

- Calories (if your dietitian or surgeon gives you a daily goal)
- Grams of protein (65 to 85 per day)
- Grams of fiber (25 to 35 per day)
- Milligrams of sodium (less than 2,300 per day)
- Certain vitamins and minerals, such as calcium and iron

Get Enough Protein!

When we ask bariatric surgery patients about the single most important dietary consideration, the most common response we hear is *"Protein!"* Most surgeons recommend at least 65 to 85 grams of protein per day. Preventing deficiency reduces muscle wasting, hair loss (alopecia), and weakness as you lose weight after surgery. Protein also helps you lose weight because it keeps you full for longer than carbohydrates or protein. Protein is so important that you should eat it first at each meal and snack.

Lean protein sources are better choices, because they are lower in calories and usually higher in other nutrients. Fatty protein sources can be high in calories and artery-clogging saturated fat.

Figure 11 – Choose lean proteins

Yes	No
fish, eggs, low-fat cheese, no-fat milk, yogurt, Greek yogurt, fat-free cottage cheese or ricotta, lean meat, shellfish, beans, skinless chicken, lean ground turkey, meat substitutes, lean low-sodium turkey or ham deli slices, beef top, bottom or eye of round roast or steak, beef sirloin steak, beef labeled "select" or "choice"	ribs, steaks (fatty), full-fat cheese, chicken with skin, ground beef, sausage, hot dogs, pepperoni, salami, bologna and other processed meats, "prime" beef, veal, fried chicken, chicken nuggets, fried fish and shrimp

Be sure to choose healthy preparation methods for your lean protein. These tips can help you keep calories down and stick to your dietary guidelines.

- ☐ Instead of frying your food, use low-fat or fat-free cooking methods such as roasting and braising. Trim off visible fat and skin.
- ☐ Keep your meat moist by using mustard, salsa, a yogurt-based marinade, or another low-calorie sauce.
- ☐ Find low-fat substitutes for unhealthy favorites such as **oven-baked chicken, egg salad** and **meatloaf**.
- ☐ Avoid adding high-calorie sauces and dressings such as mayonnaise, cheese or cream sauce, or high-sugar marinades or barbecue sauce.

Quick High-Protein Snacks

To hit your protein goals, aim for at least 10 to 20 grams of protein at each meal and snack. If you're having only three meals per day with no snacks, each meal should have about 25 grams of protein. You can get enough protein quickly by using the following ideas for snacks or small meals, and try the variations in the right-hand column; each provides at least 10 g protein. Many more snack and meal ideas are listed in the Meal Plans section.

Figure 12 – Quick high-protein snacks

Snack	Protein and Calories	Change it up! (Calorie & protein totals may change)
½ cup fat-free cottage cheese with ½ cup blueberries	15 g protein, 150 calories	Try another kind of berry or other cut fruits. Add lemon juice or cinnamon to the cottage cheese.
½ cup canned low-sodium fat-free refried beans, with 1 oz. of shredded fat-free cheddar cheese	15 g protein, 150 calories	Try this with another kind of bean, such as garbanzo, black, or pinto. Flavor the beans with diced green onions, cilantro, and/or garlic
Smoothie with 1 tbsp. peanut butter, ½ cup fat-free no-sugar-added vanilla yogurt (or plain yogurt), and ½ cup light silken tofu	14 g protein, 200 calories	Use fat-free flavored yogurt Add ½ banana or ½ cup frozen berries or peaches
1 small (5 or 6 oz.) container plain fat-free Greek yogurt with 6 whole-wheat tortilla chips	19 g protein, 160 calories	Turn the Greek yogurt into a dip with a **Greek Yogurt Dip**
Deli roll-up with 2 oz. low-fat turkey ham and 2 slices of fat-free cheese and 1 cup raw veggies	18 g protein, 170 calories	Choices include broccoli, grape tomatoes, cucumbers, celery, and bell peppers. Lap-band patients may not tolerate raw vegetables with strings or seeds. Choose any deli meat that is at least 96% fat-free, such as turkey or chicken breast or lean ham or roast beef
2 oz. canned light tuna in water or its own juice with ½ whole-wheat mini bagel (130 calories)	16 g protein, 130 calories	Try it with **tuna salad**
2 hard-boiled eggs	13 g protein, 155 calories	Slice egg whites onto a bed of spinach or other greens, or make **egg salad**.
2 large brown rice cakes with 1 oz. beef jerky	16 g protein, 160 calories	Swap the rice cakes for a low-fat cheese stick for a lower-carb higher-protein option
1 cup edamame (green soybeans) in pods with 2 tbsp. hummus	13 g protein, 200 calories	Try different flavors of hummus to vary this snack.

Protein Supplements

Many bariatric surgery patients have trouble getting enough protein. If you are not meeting your requirements, **protein shakes**, bars, or powders can help. Choose low-fat low-sugar options to limit the calories and prevent dumping syndrome (for RYGB patients).

Ask your surgeon or dietitian before using protein supplements. They can go over your diet with you to figure out how you can add more protein from food sources so you do not need supplements. If you do need extra protein, many nutritionists suggest avoiding or limiting protein shakes because they are liquids and do not satisfy hunger as well as solid foods—but you can use protein powder in shakes and other recipes, such as **Protein French Toast**.

Supplements should have at least 8 grams of protein and no more than 3 grams of sugar per 100 calories. Other options are supplements with added vitamins and minerals that are low in saturated fat. The following tables provide examples of protein supplements that meet these recommendations, and many more name-brand and store-brand options are likely available at your local supplement store or supermarket. If you make a shake with protein powder and fat-free milk, remember to add the 90 calories and 8 grams of protein per 8 oz. cup milk to your total.

Figure 13 – Protein bars

Product	Protein	Calories	Sugar	Notes
Bariatrix Proti-Bar	15 g	150	5 g	Contains 6 g sugar alcohols
Detour Lower Sugar Whey Protein	15 g	170	2 g	Contains 14 g sugar alcohols and 3.5 g saturated fat
Doctor's Carbrite Diet	21 g	190	0 g	Contains 19 g sugar alcohols
Genisoy Protein Crunch	15 g	150	1 g	Contains 13 g sugar alcohols
Glenny's Slim-Carb	12 g	130	2 g	A smaller bar you can eat with fruit or a vegetable for a more filling snack.
Labrada Hi-Protein Meal Replacement	25 g	310	7 g	Have ½ or ¼ of the bar at one time instead of the whole thing.
Medifast Crunch Bar	11 g	110	2 g	Also a good source of calcium
NuGo Smarte Carb	16 g	160	0 g	Has 7 g fiber!
Nutrilite XS Power Nutrition Energy Bar	15 g	180	3 g	Has 3 g saturated fat
Premier Nutrition Protein Eight	30 g	280	2 g	Have ½ or ¼ of the bar at one time instead of the whole thing.
Pure Protein	19 g	190	2 g	Good source of calcium
Revival Soy Smart Carb	20 g	240	2 g	Has 5 g fiber

Figure 14 – Protein shakes and powders

Product	Protein per Serving	Calories	Sugar	Notes
Unjury (powder)	21 g	100	3 g	Make with milk for 180 calories and 29 g protein or use unflavored option in soups
Glucerna Hunger smart	15 g	180	6 g	Provides fiber
Carb Solutions	21 g	110	1 g	Low-fat and high-calcium
Body Fortress	30 g	140	0	Low-fat
Muscle Milk Light Protein Shake	20 g	160	0 g	High-fiber and also comes in a 100-calorie version with 15 g protein.
Dry skim milk (powder) (1 oz.)	10 g	100	15 g	Sugars are natural in milk
Slim-Fast Lower Carb	20 g	180	1 g	Fortified with vitamins and minerals
EAS Myoplex Lite	20 g	170	4 g	High in calcium
Carnation Instant Breakfast – No Sugar Added	5 g	60	8 g	Sugars are natural milk sugars, not added sugar
Atkins Advantage Shake	15 g	160	1 g	High in fat
Designer Whey powder	18 g	100	2 g	Fortified with vitamins and minerals
Isopure Zero Carb	25	100	0	Fortified with vitamins and minerals

Protein Powder Tips and Recipes

After your post-surgery liquid diet, you might not be depending much on protein supplement. However, your dietitian might suggest them to boost your intake. The trick to using protein powders effectively is making sure that you don't add loads of calories to your diet. Consider:

- ✓ Adding them to skim milk to make high-protein shakes
- ✓ Adding them to calorie-free beverages such as hot coffee, tea, or broth
- ✓ Using them in recipes such as **pancakes** and **muffins**
- ✓ Adding them to oatmeal, cold cereal, applesauce, yogurt, dips, and puréed cooked vegetables including cauliflower and winter squash.
- ✓ Experimenting with extracts such as vanilla, mint, and almond for calorie-free flavoring
- ✓ Using unsweetened cocoa and sugar-free syrups to enhance flavor

Avoid:

- X Adding sugar to your smoothies and other protein powder recipes.
- X Choosing fruit juices often (milk and water are better choices).
- X Choosing protein powder instead of healthy, naturally high-protein foods

You Need at Least 64 oz. Fluids Each Day

Water makes up more than half the average adult's body weight. It allows your body to transport nutrients, eliminate toxins, and maintain blood pressure and body temperature. Even mild dehydration can lead to headaches, sleepiness, and muscle cramps. You need at least 64 oz. fluid each day, or eight 8-oz. cups. You need more if you sweat heavily, if the weather is warm, or if you have a fever. This is how to measure your fluid intake:

- A gallon container, half full
- Eight 8-oz. glasses
- Four half-liter water bottles
- One 2-liter bottle
- One half-gallon milk carton

After weight loss surgery, you're not allowed to drink liquids while you're eating or within 30 minutes before or after you eat solid food. If you consume fluids and solid foods together, you risk stretching your stoma (AGB), your stomach pouch (RYGB), or your gastric sleeve (VSG). Also, adding liquids to your food can make your stoma, pouch, or sleeve empty faster—so you do not stay full for long after your meal.

Getting enough water is challenging for many WLS patients. The sample schedule in the Meal Plans section shows how you can consume your 64 oz. without interfering with your meals and snacks.

Tips for Meeting Your Fluid Needs

- Set your phone or a timer to remind you each time you're supposed to drink 8 oz.
- Make a checklist of your 8 cups water, and check each one off as you drink it.
- Keep a water bottle with you at your desk, in your car, and in your gym bag.
- Drink an extra cup water before and after exercising, and every 15 to 30 minutes during exercise.
- Keep a pitcher of water in the fridge so you see it when you open the fridge.
- Many surgeons recommend that you do not use a straw because you will take in more air, which can make you feel gassy or bloated.

I Can't Drink That Much Water! What Should I Do?

After weight loss surgery, many patients find that they do not enjoy—or even cannot stand!—drinking water, even if they liked water before surgery. Luckily, you have plenty of other options to help you meet your daily fluid goals if you do not like water or if you just want some variety. One possibility is to jazz up your water!

- Try ice water—surprisingly, ice cubes in chilled water can make the water more drinkable than water without ice.
- Add a few sprigs or leaves of fresh herbs to cold water about 30 minutes before drinking it. Mint, basil, rosemary, thyme, and parsley are in the produce sections of most supermarkets; lemongrass is available in most Asian markets.

- ☐ Add a few drops of juice from a citrus fruit to your water or place a wedge of fruit on the edge of your water glass. Try lemon, lime, grapefruit, and tangerine. If you have the lap-band or are still in the liquid or puréed foods phase of your post-surgery diet progression, be careful not to get any pulp from the fruit. You can also purchase lime juice or lemon juice, often available in the baking aisle or produce section of the grocery store, instead of using fresh fruit.
- ☐ Wash, peel, and slice fresh ginger into your water about 30 minutes before drinking.
- ☐ Wash, peel, and slice fresh cucumber into your water with a leaf of bruised mint.
- ☐ Place strawberry slices or pineapple wedges on the rim of your glass.
- ☐ Freeze berries or cubes of peach in ice cube trays to add to your water.
- ☐ Use a "channel tool" to make curled lemon (or lime or orange) twists for your water.
- ☐ Add a low-calorie flavored beverage powder such as Crystal Light to your water.
- ☐ Add a few drops of vanilla extract and a packet of low-calorie sugar substitute.

If you just can't face water, you have plenty of other options. Keep them low-calorie or calorie-free, and avoid carbonated beverages such as soft drinks and sparkling waters.

- ☐ Decaffeinated instant or brewed coffee.
- ☐ Make hot tea with decaffeinated black, green, or white tea or herbal tea bags or instant powder—just be sure to choose sugar-free or unsweetened instant powders.
- ☐ Make hot tea with a twist of orange peel and a dash of cinnamon.
- ☐ Try hot tea with a spoonful of blackberry juice or Crystal Light added.
- ☐ Try cooling and refrigerating hot tea and then adding ice just before serving.
- ☐ Unsweetened or diet ready-to-drink iced tea (check the caffeine content).
- ☐ Choose ready-to-drink, non-carbonated, flavored sugar-free beverages such as flavored waters, diet lemonade, or diet fruit-flavored drinks.
- ☐ Low-sodium bouillon
- ☐ Sugar-free gelatin
- ☐ Sugar-free ice pops

List of Name Brands with Low-Calorie Beverages

Each of these choices has 10 or fewer calories per 8-oz. (1-cup) serving.

- ☐ Nestea diet and unsweetened iced teas
- ☐ Crystal Light
- ☐ Snapple diet juice drinks and teas
- ☐ Fuze Slenderize beverages
- ☐ Lipton diet or unsweetened
- ☐ Ocean-Spray diet drinks (avoid the "light" ones, with 50 calories per 1-cup serving)
- ☐ Sugar-free Kool-Aid
- ☐ Arizona sugar-free stix and powdered mix and diet iced tea
- ☐ Welch's diet juice drinks
- ☐ Langer's H2O 0 Calories Vitamin Enhanced Water (some flavors are 50 calories per serving)

Keep It Low-Calorie: Beverages versus Foods

Keep your beverages calorie-free or low-calorie, with no more than 10 calories per 8-oz. (1-cup) serving. “Drinking your calories” is one of the easiest, fastest ways to make your surgery ineffective. Fluids go through your stomach pouch or sleeve quickly, and they are less filling than solid foods. The table below compares some beverages with examples of nutritious foods that contain the same number of calories. Choosing solid foods helps with weight loss.

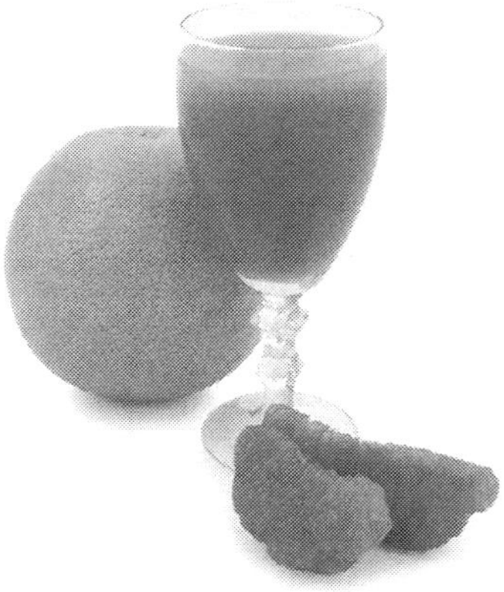

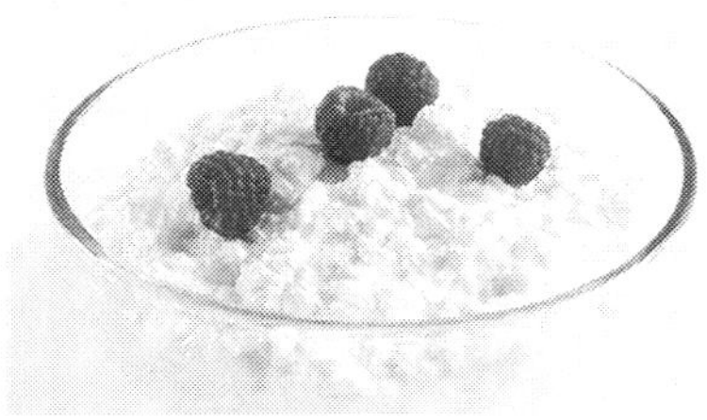

100 calories: 1 cup grapefruit juice versus ½ cup nonfat cottage cheese

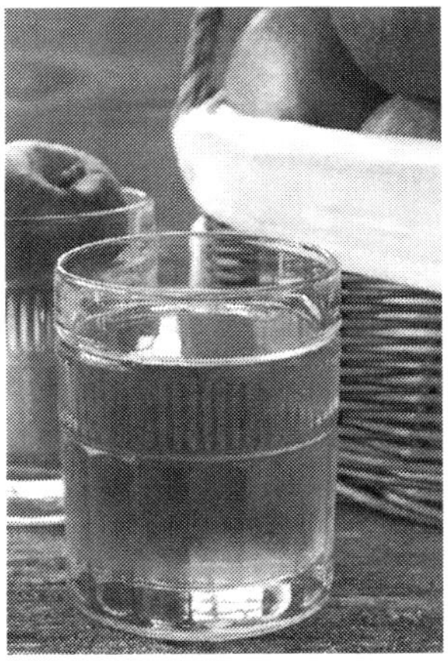

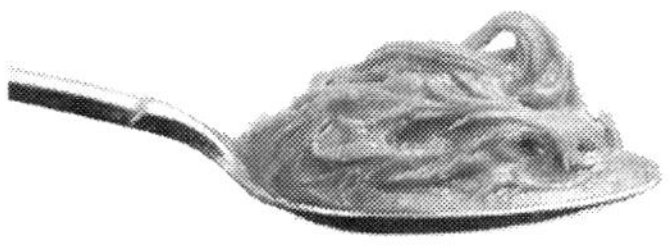

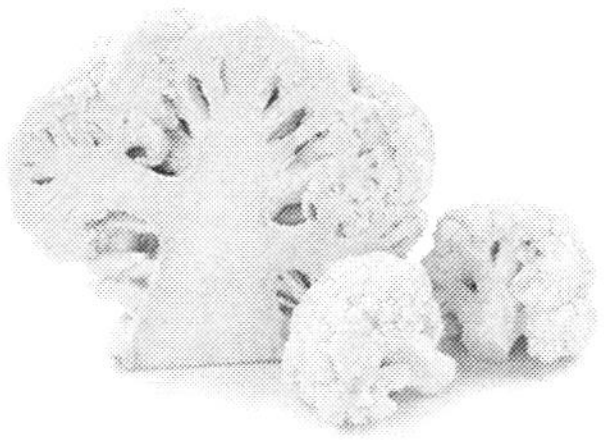

120 calories: 1 cup apple juice versus 1 tbsp. peanut butter plus 1 cup cauliflower florets

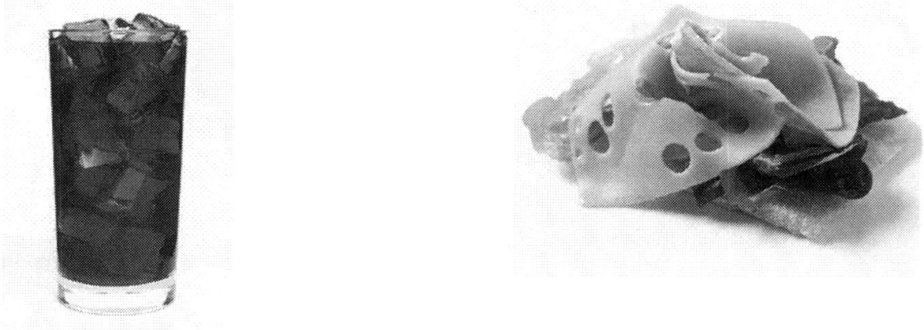

140 calories: 1 cup cranberry juice versus 2 oz. turkey ham plus 1 oz. low-fat cheese

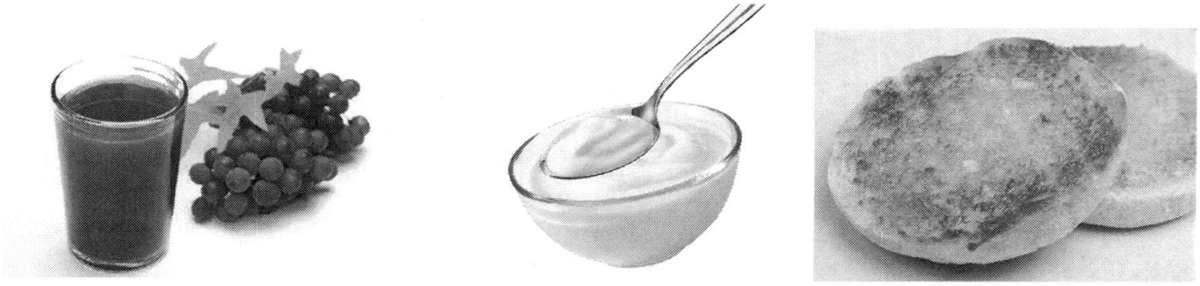

160 calories: 1 cup grape juice versus 5 oz. non-fat plain Greek yogurt plus ½ English muffin

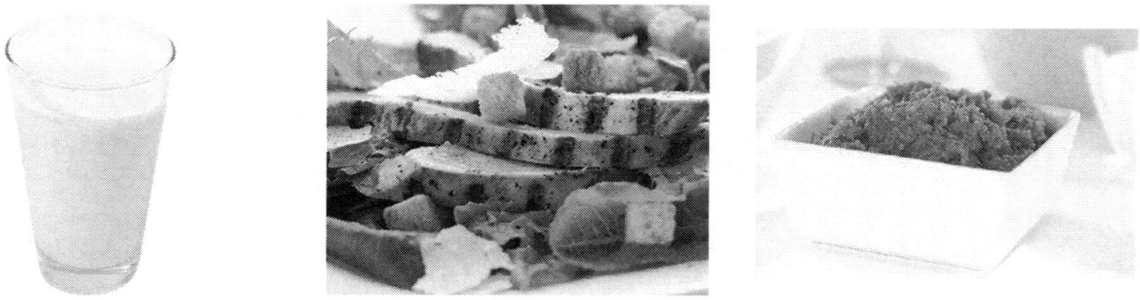

190 calories: 10 oz. (1 can) Special K protein shake versus 3 oz. grilled chicken plus ½ cup mashed sweet potato

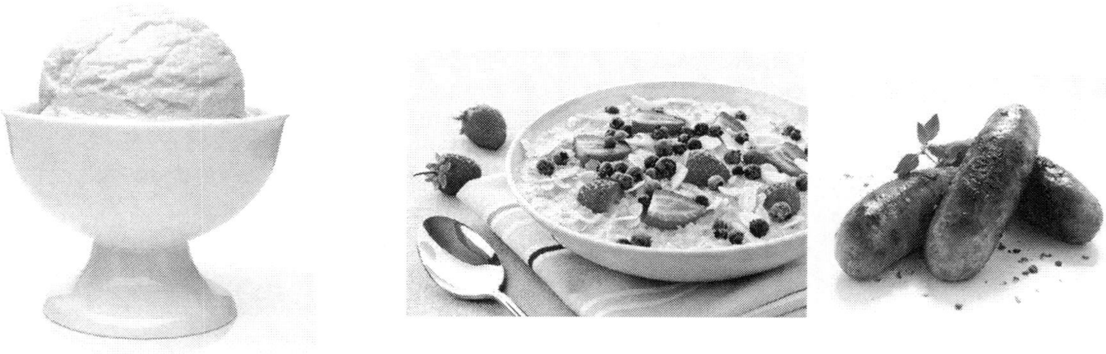

260 calories: ½ cup regular ice cream versus 1 packet instant oatmeal plus 1 cup melon or berries, plus 2 lean turkey breakfast links

Sometimes you may need to drink calorie-containing beverages. High-protein options such as milk and protein shakes may be appropriate under the following circumstances.

- In your post-surgery diet progression, on a liquid diet or puréed foods diet
- When you need extra protein and cannot get it from foods. Vertical sleeve patients are most likely to encounter this situation regularly, even long after surgery.
- When you are experiencing complications from your procedure and are having trouble with solid food.
- If you are a lap-band patient, in the days following a band fill, because you may be sensitive to solid foods.
- Any time your surgeon or nutritionist recommends such beverages

Caffeine After Weight Loss Surgery

Many surgeons recommend limiting or avoiding caffeine after weight loss surgery. Caffeine's acidity can irritate your stomach and increase your risk of gastroesophageal reflux disease (GERD) and heartburn, especially with AGB. It can also reduce your body's ability to absorb nutrients such as iron and calcium. Weight loss surgery already puts you at risk for deficiencies of these nutrients, and caffeine can exacerbate this.

Consume caffeine only if your surgeon or dietitian allows you to, and consume only the recommended amount. That may be about one cup coffee per day. Avoid high-calorie caffeinated pitfalls such as hot chocolate with milk and sugar, sweetened iced teas, and milk-based or sugar-sweetened bottled and coffee shop coffee beverages such as lattes, mochas, and frappuccinos. Common sources of caffeine include:

- Coffee
- Coffee-containing foods such as coffee ice cream and candy
- Hot chocolate
- Chocolate and chocolate-containing foods
- Green and black tea
- Energy drinks

What About Alcohol After WLS?

Alcohol provides calories without protein or other important nutrients, and it can increase your risk of ulcers. Drinking alcohol can further derail your weight loss because it relaxes you. When you drink, you are less likely to stick to your meal plan and resist high-calorie foods. Furthermore, drinking on an empty stomach lowers your alcohol tolerance, but drinking while you eat solid foods goes against WLS dietary guidelines.

If your doctor approves alcohol, stay within the standard recommendations of a daily maximum of one drink for women and two drinks for men. A drink is:

- 12 oz. beer (150 calories)
- 5 oz. wine (120 calories)
- 1.5 oz. hard liquor (120 calories)
- Mixed drinks (200 or more calories, including sugar)

Kitchen: What You Need

Make sure your kitchen is stocked with these things *before* you go to the hospital.

Figure 15 – Pre-surgery grocery list

Grocery Item	Servings / Pkg	Serv Size	Cal/ Serv	g Pro/ Serv
MEAT/MEAT SUBSTITUTE				
14 oz container *Nasoya Extra Firm* Tofu	3	5 oz	120	14
24 oz container *Market Pantry* Fat Free Cottage Cheese	6	½ c	70	11
20 oz package *Jenny-O* Extra Lean Ground Turkey Breast (99/1)	10	2 oz	60	13
8 oz container *Archer Farms* Grilled Chicken Strips	4	2 oz	80	14
9 oz container *Oscar Mayer Oven Roasted Deli Turkey*	5	6 slices	45	8
12 oz bag *Market Pantry* Lite Mozzarella String Cheese	12	1 stick	60	8
24 oz bag *Market Pantry* Frozen Tilapia	12	2 oz (½ filet)	45	10
1 dozen *Sunups* Grade A, Large Eggs	12	1 egg	70	6
4.5 oz package *Starkist Tuna Creations* (zesty lemon pepper or hickory smoked)	2	2 oz	60	14
DAIRY/DAIRY SUBSTITUTE				
32 oz container *Chobani* Plain, Nonfat Greek Yogurt	8	½ c	70	11
1 gallon *Market Pantry* Skim Milk	16	1 c	90	8

credit: Medical University of South Carolina weight loss surgery program

Kitchen Aids

- ☐ 1 set of measuring cups
- ☐ 1 set of measuring spoons (likely on a ring through holes in the handles)
- ☐ Digital or analog kitchen scale
- ☐ A cute set of small dishes to help you eat smaller portions
- ☐ A cute set of kid-sized silverware to help you eat more slowly
- ☐ Standard or immersion blender (for smoothies, shakes, puréed foods)
- ☐ Small containers with tight-fitting lids, zip bags to help you transport food or store it in the fridge or freezer
- ☐ Insulated lunch bag
- ☐ Reusable water bottle and insulated spill-proof travel mug
- ☐ Ice cube trays
- ☐ Oil spritzer for low-calorie cooking and salad dressings

Refrigerator

- ☐ Beverages
  - Water pitcher (with or without flavorings or teas)
  - Teas, anything you've prepared (flavored water)
  - Fat-free milk
- ☐ Lean protein
  - Eggs or liquid egg whites
  - Deli meats: ham, turkey, chicken breast slices or vegetarian slices
  - Fresh lean meat and poultry, seafood
  - Lean turkey or vegetarian bacon or breakfast sausage
- ☐ Dairy
  - Fat-free yogurt or Greek yogurt, plain or flavored with no added sugar
  - String cheese
  - Low-fat or fat-free brick or shredded cheese, low-fat parmesan
  - Fat-free cottage cheese
  - Fat-free ricotta cheese
  - Laughing Cow light cheese
- ☐ Fresh veggies
  - Bagged salad mix, spinach, or mixed greens, or head of lettuce
  - For snacking: baby carrots, grape tomatoes, broccoli and cauliflower florets, cucumber
  - For cooking: any fresh whole vegetables or pre-cut vegetables, such as soup mix, broccoli florets, stir fry mix
- ☐ Fresh fruit
  - Whole fruit such as apples, oranges, berries, grapes
  - Pre-cut melons
- ☐ Starches
  - High-fiber whole-grain wraps, tortillas, or pita pockets
  - Low-calorie sliced bread (less than 50 calories per slice)
  - Sweet potatoes
- ☐ Condiments
  - Peanut butter
  - Hummus
  - Low-calorie or fat-free salad dressing
  - Light soy sauce, Worcestershire sauce
  - Tran- fat-free margarine spread
  - Yellow, deli, or Dijon mustard

Pantry

- ☐ Beverages
  - Decaffeinated green, black, or herbal tea bags or loose tea or powder
  - Instant or ground decaffeinated coffee
  - Diet cocoa mix
- ☐ Protein
  - Canned (or pouched) tuna in water or its own juice

  - Other canned proteins such as salmon, mackerel, shrimp, and chicken
  - Canned beans, fat-free refried beans, and lentils
  - Shelf-stable tofu
- ☐ Vegetables
  - Canned tomatoes, tomato paste, tomato sauce (all are great for cooking)
  - Any canned vegetable, such as artichoke hearts, green beans, carrots, spinach
- ☐ Fruit
  - Applesauce
  - Pure pumpkin purée (*not* pumpkin pie filling)
  - Any fruit canned in its own juice or fruit cups without added sugar
- ☐ Starches and Snacks
  - Oatmeal, unflavored or sugar-free
  - High-fiber breakfast cereal such as Fiber One
  - Dried barley, brown rice, and any other whole grain
  - Whole-grain pasta
  - Rice cakes, whole grain crackers, and pretzel sticks
  - Roasted nuts and peanuts
  - Trail mix
  - Popcorn (not lap-band) – low-fat microwave or plain kernels
- ☐ Baking/cooking
  - Savory and sweet spices such as ground black pepper, cumin, curry powder, basil, oregano, cinnamon, ginger, cloves, and nutmeg
  - Calorie-free sweetener (sugar substitute), such as stevia (Truvia), sucralose (Splenda), aspartame (Equal) and saccharin (Sweet 'n' Low)
  - Olive oil, vegetable oil (canola, sunflower, safflower)
  - Fat-free cooking spray
- ☐ Meal aids and condiments
  - Spaghetti sauce
  - Low-fat low-sodium chunky broth-based soup, such as vegetable beef (add protein powder)
  - Low-sodium bouillon/broth for cooking
  - Seasoning packets such as for tacos or chili
  - Salad dressing mix for salad dressings and dips
  - Vinegar (white, red wine, balsamic, and rice)
  - Fat-free mayonnaise
- ☐ Dietary supplements: vitamin, mineral, omega-3 fatty acid and other supplements you take

Freezer

- ☐ Protein
  - Veggie burgers
  - Frozen chicken breasts, turkey burgers, ready-to-cook shrimp, other lean proteins
  - Beans or green soybeans (edamame)
- ☐ Vegetables
  - Peas, mixed vegetables, corn, broccoli, spinach, zucchini and yellow squash
  - Winter squash or vegetables in low-fat sauce

- Fruit
    - Unsweetened (no sugar added) berries, mango, melon, and pineapple, and fruit salads
    - Fruit juice pops (homemade or storebought)
- Split whole-grain low-calorie English muffins and mini bagels
- Frozen low-calorie, high-protein lunches and dinners with lean protein (such as chicken breast, sirloin, or shrimp), a nutritious starch (such as brown rice, whole wheat pasta, or sweet potatoes), and a serving of vegetables.
    - Lean meals from Lean Cuisine, Kashi, Healthy Choice, Michelina's Lean Gourmet, and Weight Watcher's Smart Ones often meet these requirements.
- Frozen low-calorie, high-protein breakfasts such as egg white and turkey sausage sandwiches on an English muffin or whole-grain bagel, or egg white omelets with vegetables.

Keep Measuring Your Food!

Measuring your food is a powerful weapon when your bathroom scale seems to be plotting against you. As they get further out from surgery, many weight loss surgery patients stop measuring their food because constantly using measuring cups and spoons and food scales can be tiresome. They think they can judge their hunger and fullness on their own, or they think they can "eyeball" their portion sizes instead of measuring them. Don't make these mistakes!

Weight, in ounces or grams, is the most accurate measurement for most foods. It's especially useful for meat, poultry and fish, dry pasta, oatmeal and rice, nuts and peanuts, fresh fruits and vegetables, bread that wasn't pre-sliced, breakfast cereals and cheese.

Like bathroom scales, kitchen (food) scales can be mechanical with a dial, or digital with an electronic reading.

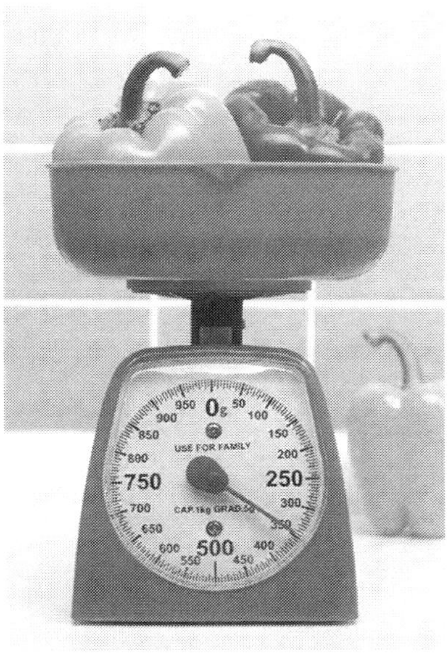

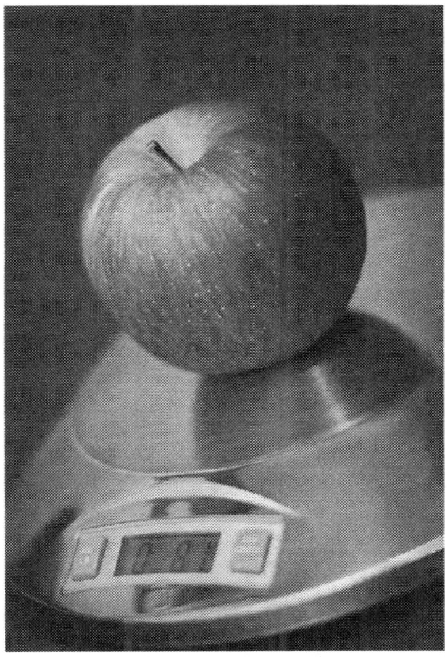

Here's how to determine the weight of a portion of food, for example, the weight of a chicken breast:

1. Turn the scale on (digital).
2. On the scale, place the (empty) dish that you will be using for your food. Many scales come with their own bowl. You can use that one or your own.
3. "Tare" the scale by setting the needle to the "0" mark (mechanical) or by pressing the tare button (digital).
4. Place the portion of food in the bowl.
5. Read the weight by looking at the needle (mechanical) or by noting the number on the scale's screen (digital).

To serve yourself a predetermined weight of food, for example 1 oz. of macaroni from a large box, follow steps 1-3 above and then slowly add macaroni to the bowl until you reach the proper weight of the food serving. Don't forget to check whether your scale is displaying grams or ounces!

Measuring Food Volume

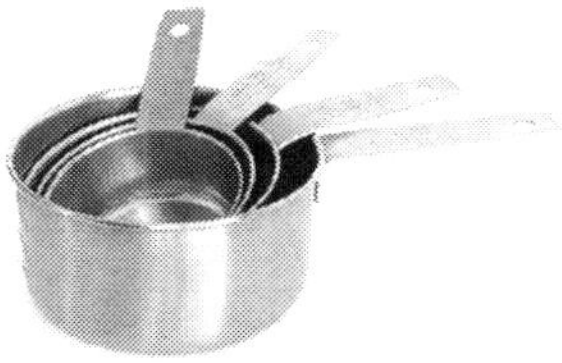

You can also measure food volume, in units of fluid ounces, cups, and tablespoons. This can be useful for cooked grains and vegetables, cut raw vegetables and fruits, berries, yogurt and milk, peanut butter, hummus, oils, soup, salad dressing, and soy sauce.

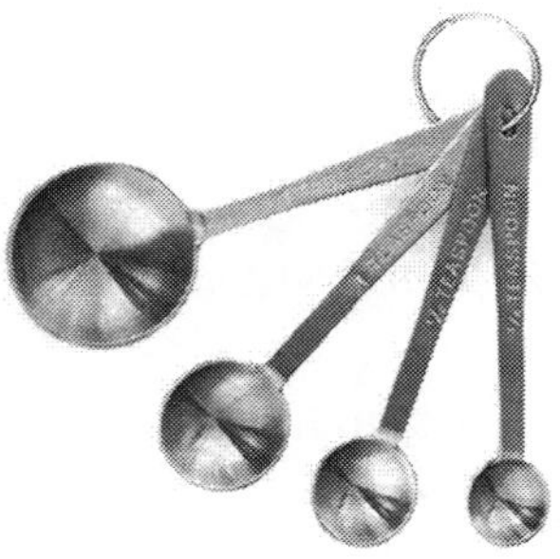

Your kitchen should have a set of measuring spoons and measuring cups and a heat-resistant glass measuring cup with marks on the side for measuring liquids. Specialty home and kitchen stores sell them, and you can buy inexpensive sets at most supermarkets, drugstores or even dollar stores. Many foods can be measured using weight *or* volume *or* by counting. The important thing is to measure *everything* to monitor what you are eating!

Help with Measurements

Fluid ounces, cups, and tablespoons may seem complicated, but these conversions can become automatic with practice. The table below shows some common conversions.

Figure 16 – Conversion Table for Measuring Volume

Unit	Equals	Also Equals:	Examples
1 tsp.	⅓ tbsp.	5 milliliters (5 ml)	1 tsp. margarine or olive oil
1 tbsp.	3 tsp.	½ fluid oz. (15 ml)	1 tbsp. peanut butter
2 tbsp.	1/8 cup	1 fl. oz. (30 ml)	2 tbsp. hummus
4 tbsp.	¼ cup	2 fl. oz. (60 ml)	¼ cup protein powder, cheese
8 tbsp.	½ cup	4 fl. oz. (120 ml)	½ cup cooked green beans
16 tbsp.	1 cup	8 fl. oz. (240 ml)	1 cup cereal or yogurt
2 cups	1 pint	16 fl. oz. (480 ml or nearly ½ liter)	1 bottle of water
4 cups	1 quart	32 fl. oz. (960 ml or just under 1 liter)	1 quart of soup (freeze in four servings)

Real Life: Measuring!

Sometimes you simply cannot measure your portions. You might, for example, eat at a restaurant or find yourself at work without a scale or measuring cups and spoons. In these situations, visualizing objects can help you estimate proper portion sizes.

The table below shows some handy estimates. Remember to use these estimates only when necessary; when you can, measure your food precisely!

Figure 17 – Food servings and similarly-sized objects

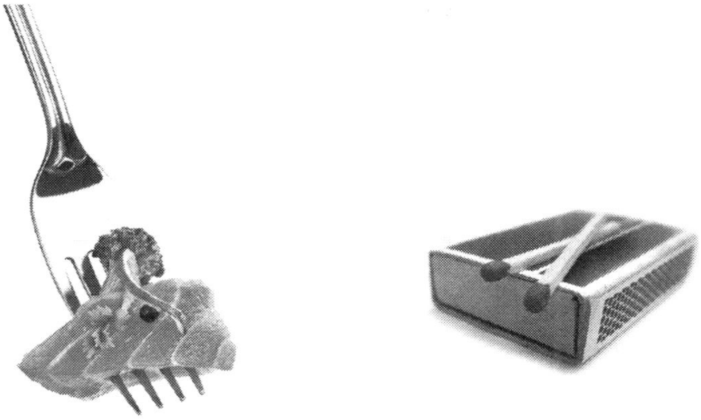

1 oz. meat or fish = 1 matchbox

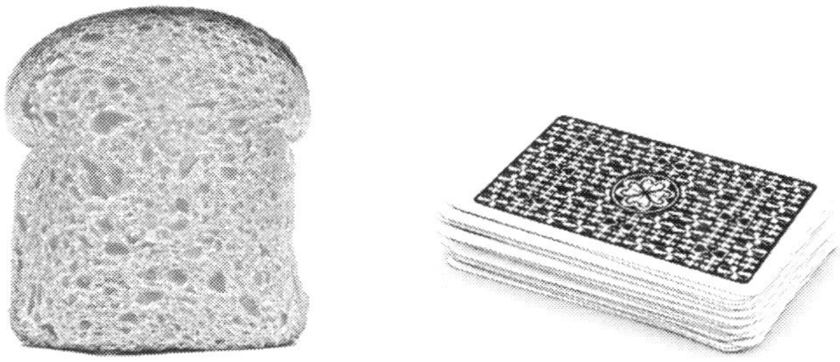

3 oz. meat OR a 1-oz. slice of bread = deck of cards

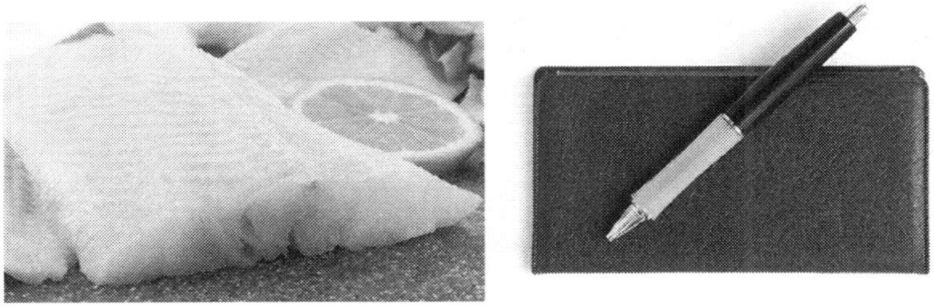

3 oz. fish = a checkbook

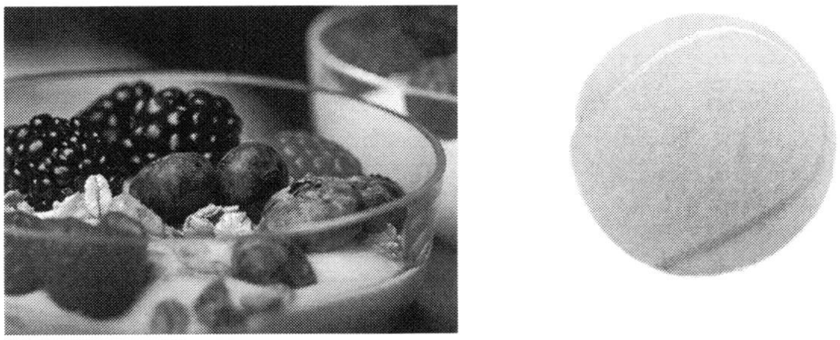

1 medium apple OR 1 cup cereal, fruit, or pasta = a tennis ball

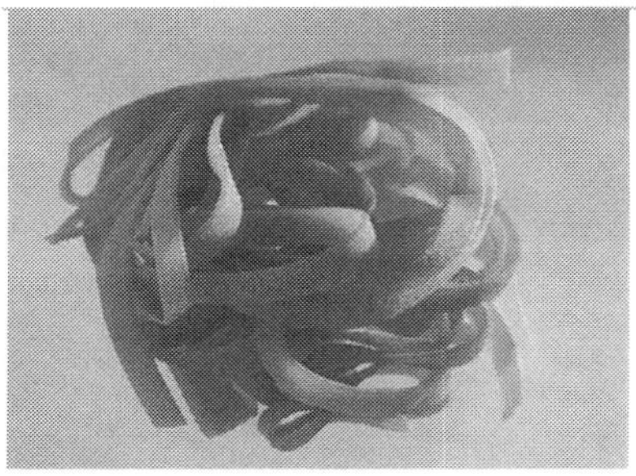

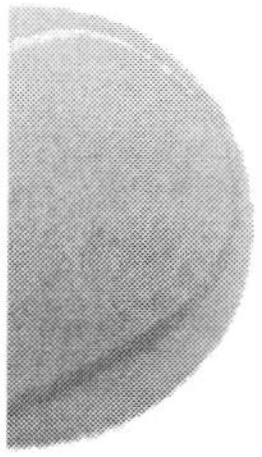

½ cup dry pasta = ½ tennis ball

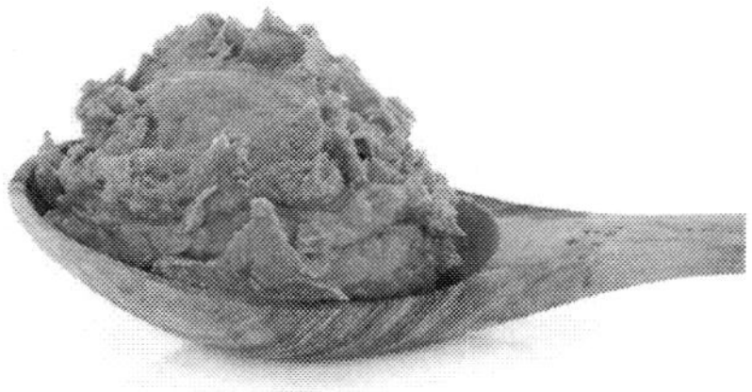

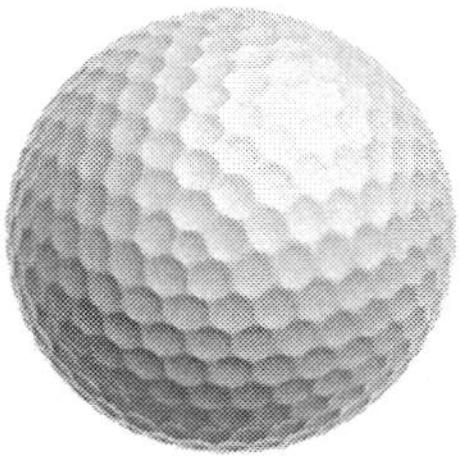

2 tbsp. peanut butter = a golf ball

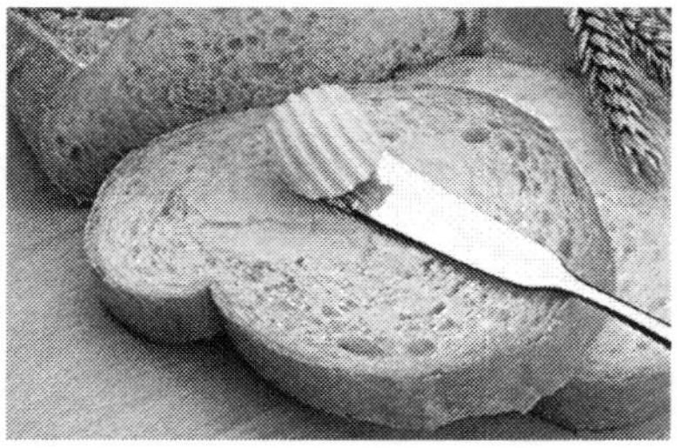

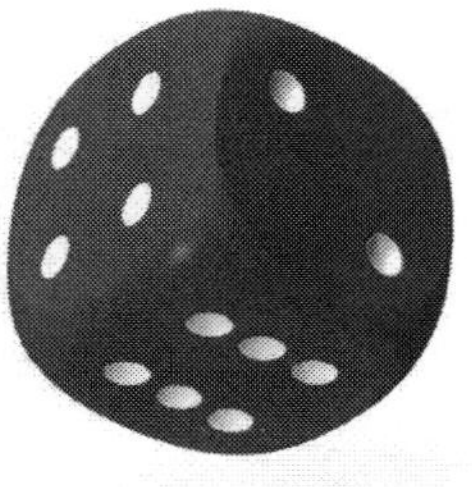

1 tsp. butter or margarine or oil = 1 die

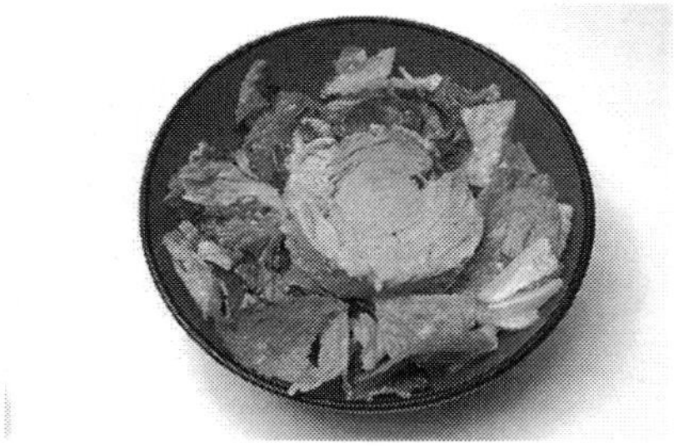

¼ cup tuna = 1 egg

Where Does the Time Go??

Eating right, exercising, and staying positive are easier when you have plenty of time, but all of us are limited to 24 hours per day. As a weight loss surgery patient, you have the same responsibilities as anyone else, *plus* the extra obligations of taking care of your diet and workouts. These tips can help you make the most of your 24 hours a day and seven days a week.

Prioritize: Budgeting your time is like budgeting your money—you start with the essentials and finish with the luxuries. For money, you might start with groceries and shelter, and finish by dedicating leftover money to a vacation fund. Non-negotiable priorities include:

- Sleep
- Work (including commute time)
- Family obligations such as childcare
- Personal obligations such as doctor appointments

Less rigid priorities can be modified. You can cut back on them or change the time that you do them. They include:

- Religious services
- Church groups and other social clubs
- Leisure and fun time for hobbies
- Household chores and errands
- Family time

Your health priorities are the ones you have to fit into your schedule. They include:

- Food preparation
- Eating time for 3 to 6 meals or snacks per day
- Food planning once a week or every day
- Food logging, every day or after each meal
- Grocery shopping, usually two or more times per week
- Support group meetings
- Exercise

Time-Saving Tips: With some creativity, you can multitask or use other time-saving strategies to organize your priorities and leave time for optional parts of your schedule.

- Turn chores and errands into family time. Instead of feeling like you wasted an hour cleaning the house and making dinner, you will find that the hour flies by and you are now caught up on your family's interests and activities.
- Get some quality weekend time with your spouse or a good friend by asking them to help you prepare your food during your weekly session (see the Plan your Meals section). If the two of you eat different foods because of your WLS diet, offer to help prepare their foods for the week—or have a shared cooking day!
- Instead of meeting your friends for lunch, ask them to meet you for a fun workout like a walk or hike or a shared picnic.

- ☐ Always have something to do while you're waiting. For example, plan or log your meals on your smartphone while waiting in line or for the bus or a doctor's appointment.
- ☐ Keep sturdy walking shoes in your car, and in winter, extra layers of clothing. Walk briskly when your child's activities run late or when you're waiting on a car repair.
- ☐ Shower at the gym so you don't have to come back home before work.
- ☐ Have your children carpool to school—you'll be driving only one-half or one-third the time you did before. This strategy also helps you meet parents who could care for your children when you need some time to yourself.

Plan: You will get the most out of your days when you plan what you are going to do. Try filling out a typical weekly schedule using the samples below as guides.

Figure 18 – Sample weekday schedule

Time	Activity	Meals, Snacks, Fluids and Supplements
6:30 a.m.	Wake up and shower.	Drink 1 cup water
7:00 a.m.	Wake up family, pack lunches and make breakfast.	
7:30 a.m.		Breakfast with multivitamin with calcium
8:00 a.m.	Drop off children at school on way to work.	
8:30 a.m.	Arrive at work.	1 cup water
9:00 a.m.		
9:30 a.m.		1 cup water with iron and vitamin B12 supplement
10:00 a.m.	Walk or stretch on break.	Snack 1
10:30 a.m.		
11:00 a.m.		1 cup water
11:30 a.m.		
noon		Lunch with a multivitamin with calcium
12:30 p.m.	Finish lunch hour with a brisk walk.	
1:00 p.m.		1 cup water
1:30 p.m.		
2:00 p.m.		1 cup water
2:30 p.m.		
3:00 p.m.	Plan tomorrow's menu; make shopping list on break from work	Snack 2
3:30 p.m.		
4:00 p.m.		
4:30 p.m.	Leave work to pick up children.	1 cup water
5:00 p.m.	Grocery shopping or any needed errands.	
5: 30 p.m.	Make dinner.	
6:00 p.m.		Dinner with a calcium supplement
6:30 p.m.		
7:00 p.m.	Home workout DVD, walk outside or stationary bike	1 cup water
7:30 p.m.	Help children with homework	
8:00 p.m.	Plan and prepare food and workouts for tomorrow.	
8:30 p.m.		
9:00 p.m.	Put children to bed.	
9:30 p.m.	Relax.	
10:00 p.m.	Bed	

Figure 19 – Sample weekend schedule

Time	Activity	Meals, Snacks, Fluids and Supplements Weekend Day
7:00 a.m.	Wake up.	Drink 1 cup water
7:30 a.m.	Make family breakfast. Pack snack 1.	
8:00 a.m.		Breakfast with multivitamin with calcium
8:30 a.m.		
9:00 a.m.		1 cup water
9:30 a.m.	Gym. Cardio and weights.	1 cup water
10:00 a.m.		
10:30 a.m.		Snack 1 with iron and vitamin B12 supplement
11:00 a.m.	Go home. Shower.	
11:30 a.m.	Make lunch. Pack Snack 2.	1 cup water
noon	Family meal.	Lunch with a multivitamin with calcium
12:30 p.m.		
1:00 p.m.	Drive children to soccer practice. Watch while walking sidelines or around field.	1 cup water
1:30 p.m.		
2:00 p.m.	If still at practice, plan menus, log meals and make shopping lists.	1 cup water
2:30 p.m.		
3:00 p.m.	Take children home. Stop at supermarket or anywhere else necessary.	Snack 2
3:30 p.m.		
4:00 p.m.	"down" time: help children with homework, clean house, relax.	
4:30 p.m.		1 cup water
5:00 p.m.		
5: 30 p.m.	Make dinner.	
6:00 p.m.		Dinner with a calcium supplement
6:30 p.m.		
7:00 p.m.	Family time:	1 cup water
7:30 p.m.	Help children with homework	
8:00 p.m.	Plan and prepare food and workouts for tomorrow.	
8:30 p.m.		
9:00 p.m.	Put children to bed.	
9:30 p.m.	Relax.	
10:00 p.m.	Bed	

Dietary Supplements After Bariatric Surgery

A side effect of your very low-calorie diet after weight loss surgery is the high risk for nutritional deficiencies. Because you are not consuming much food, you have more trouble meeting your daily requirements for certain vitamins and minerals just from regular food sources. Roux-en-Y gastric bypass patients may need higher doses of some supplements because of nutrient malabsorption after surgery. Vertical sleeve gastrectomy patients may need to take extra supplements because of reduced stomach size. The table below lists some of the most common supplements for bariatric surgery patients.

Figure 20 – Likely supplements for weight loss surgery patients

Nutrient	Why Needed	Who's at Higher Risk
Iron	Prevent anemia	Vegetarians Women who are menstruating
Folic acid	Prevent neural tube defects (women who may become pregnant) Prevent anemia	Women who may become pregnant Non-compliance with daily multivitamin
Vitamin B12 (sublingual or injection)	Prevent anemia Support nerve function Prevent nerve damage from deficiency	Vegans (strict vegetarians) Post-surgery IBD patients (after upper bowel resection)
Calcium (calcium citrate)	Strengthen bones (prevent osteoporosis) Proper muscle and nerve function	Roux-en-Y gastric bypass patients Vertical sleeve gastrectomy patients Lactose intolerant individuals who limit dairy products
Vitamin D	Strengthen bones (prevent osteoporosis) Lower risk of other diseases, such as inflammatory bowel disease (IBD) and rheumatoid arthritis	Roux-en-Y gastric bypass patients Very low-fat diet Not drinking milk or eating oily fish such as salmon and albacore
Vitamin A	Prevent night blindness Maintain healthy skin	Roux-en-Y gastric bypass patients Very low-fat diet

Other common supplements include:

- ☐ A daily multivitamin/mineral supplement (gastric bypass patients may need two daily).
- ☐ B-complex supplement.
- ☐ Omega-3 fish oil supplement if you do not eat seafood regularly.

Your surgeon or dietitian should tell you exactly which vitamins and minerals to take. You will probably need to take them for life. Immediately after surgery, liquid supplements or crushed pills may be necessary. Later, you can try chewable tablets. You might not ever be able to swallow large pills; you may need a pill splitter or a pill crusher.

Most bariatric surgery patients do not need protein supplements, but some do. See the section on Protein for more information.

You can time your supplements to maximize the amount of nutrients you absorb. The Time Management section suggests a sample daily schedule to optimally manage your supplements. A pill organizer with separate compartments for each day of the week will help you effectively keep track of scheduled supplements for each day.

Adjustments for Lap-band Patients

The adjustable gastric band works by narrowing the opening between the top of your stomach, now the stoma, and the larger pouch that is now your lower stomach. This slows down the passage of food from the top of your stomach to the bottom pouch. When the band is fuller, it causes more restriction by narrowing the opening from the stoma to the large stomach pouch. When the band is not as full, the opening is wider and food moves more quickly to the large stomach pouch.

Your first fill—the injection of fluid into your band to increase restriction—comes about four to six weeks after surgery, when you are starting to eat solid foods. The surgeon injects fluid through your access port, which is just under the surface of your skin near your belly button. The surgeon may use a local anaesthetic to numb the area before injecting. The process is simple, and takes about 5 to 10 minutes.

With more restriction (a fuller band), the stomach takes longer to empty, so you feel full sooner and stay full for longer. This can speed up weight loss. With less restriction (a less full band), you do not fill up as fast and you get hungrier sooner because the stomach empties faster. Weight loss can therefore be slower. A band that is too full can be dangerous, though. It's important that your band is at exactly the right fill level for you.

You may need your band volume, or fill level, adjusted a few times before you get the right level. This is also known as the Green Zone, which may change over time. The figure below illustrates the different zones and how you know when you are in the Green Zone or when you need a fill or un-fill.

Figure 21 – The Green Zone

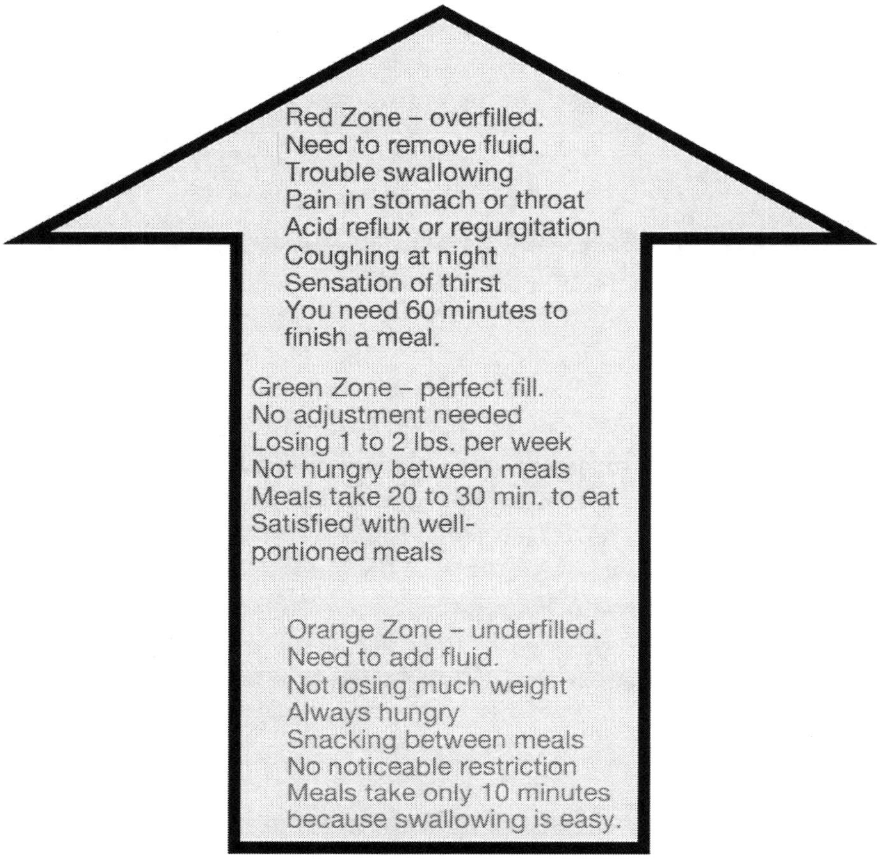

Adjustments can cause your stomach to swell and make the band feel uncomfortably tight. Because of this, you may need to change your diet after an adjustment. Do just liquid diet on the day of your adjustment. Progress to puréed or soft foods for the next day or two before gradually returning to your regular lap-band diet with solid foods. These are a few more tips for getting adjustments to work for you:

- Be cautious about pushing your doctor for fills too often. If you are not losing weight, make sure you are following the lap-band diet before asking for a fill. Remember, filling the band too full is dangerous and will not help in consistent weight loss.
- Always know how to contact the nearest available surgeon for an emergency adjustment. This includes weekend and overnight surgeons, as well as surgeons in any location where you are traveling.
- Do not schedule adjustments immediately before traveling, because you may need to return to your surgeon if the band is too tight.
- You may need to get your band completely unfilled if you are sick and are having trouble staying hydrated or nourished or if you develop esophagitis and need to allow the inflammation and pain to subside. You may also need to have it unfilled if you become pregnant.

Willpower, "Want Power" and Other Mind Games

Weight loss surgery success is not easy. You need to make the right decisions constantly.

- Add a hard-boiled egg white or bacon to your salad?
- Drink water or have a latté?
- Eat the chicken wings or order a side salad?
- Exercise or sleep in?
- Stop eating or go for seconds?

And so it goes, day after day. You need to be self-disciplined to make these good decisions consistently. Strength to resist temptations comes from motivation to succeed, from your support system, and from your fear of developing side effects or complications related to poor diet after weight loss surgery. You are not alone when you struggle to make the right decisions.

Some people see it is a question of willpower, or the ability to resist impulses. Strong willpower can help you choose healthy foods over delicious but high-calorie choices; willpower can also get you out the door for a walk instead of sitting on the couch. Willpower helps you walk past the cookies in the lunchroom at work without grabbing one. But many weight loss surgery patients get discouraged at the thought of depending on willpower because they think that theirs is not strong enough.

"Want power" is another way to consider your mental strength. While willpower focuses on your ability to resist temptation, *want power emphasizes your opportunities to decide what you want*. With want power, you are so focused on getting what you want that everything else is just a distraction. For example, you can be focused on:

- avoiding dumping syndrome so you truly have no desire to eat the fudge.
- keeping up with your best friend in an upcoming 5K road race, so you do not consider skipping your workout.
- having a good weigh-in so you do not eat a bite without measuring it first.
- showing your wife that the cost of surgery was worthwhile, so you attend all your support group meetings.
- setting a good example for your children; you are not even tempted to eat chips while watching television.

You probably already use want power in other areas of your life. For example, if you have children, you make sure they do their homework each night because your desire for them to do well in school trumps your desire to let them play video games. The decision is a no-brainer. It is not a sacrifice requiring willpower; instead, it is an easy decision with positive results of children who are better-disciplined and achieve higher grades in school.

Whether you choose to think of it as willpower, want power or even "won't power" (as in "I won't do anything that will hurt me"), practice helps. Start by getting into the habit of mentally listing the pros and cons of a choice.

For example, the pros of eating the cookie are a minute or two of pleasure, and complimenting the baker on how good the cookies are. The cons include more calories and sugar than you need, a guilty feeling that can last for hours, the risk of dumping syndrome (especially for gastric bypass patients) and losing credibility at work about your commitment to your new lifestyle—thus risking that your work colleagues will continue to offer you junk food and pressure you to accept when you refuse. When you weigh the pros and cons like this, the obvious decision is to skip the cookie.

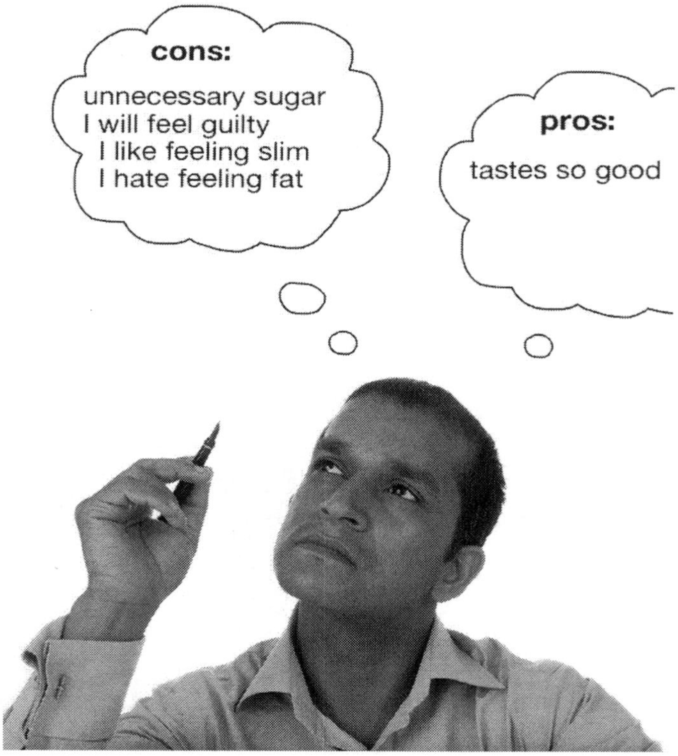

The best thing about good decisions is momentum. Getting into the groove is often harder than staying in it. Because thinking about making good decisions for the rest of your life can be daunting, a mental trick to get you started so you can build momentum is to focus on smaller chunks of time. Think about getting through the meal, then getting through the morning and through the day. Gain confidence as you go from wondering whether you *can* to knowing that you *will*.

Prepare for the Long Haul

You almost certainly tried to lose weight many times before you chose to have weight loss surgery. Some of the diets may have worked for a few weeks or months. Then you stopped following the diet and gained the weight right back. How will you make sure your weight loss surgery leads to lasting weight loss?

- ✓ Have confidence.
- ✓ Stay motivated.
- ✓ Be patient.

Confidence Takes the Doubt out of Weight Loss

When you are confident, you do not have to worry.

You can be confident that the weight loss surgery diet works. If you stick to your low-calorie, high-protein meal plan, you *will* lose weight. Trusting in your diet means that you do not have to second-guess yourself. Just follow the meal plan, and you will lose weight.

Be confident that you can do it; self-doubt is a dangerous thing. Whenever you question whether you can do something, you open yourself up to the possibility of not achieving it. Just replace your doubting thoughts with positive and confident thoughts. Don't think, "Will I eat the meals that I planned for myself?" Think instead, "It's time to finish preparing the meals that I planned for myself today." Don't think, "Will I have time to exercise today?" Think instead, "I've got my gym bag all packed and know exactly which exercises I will do at the gym on the way home from work today." These thoughts eliminate doubts about your healthy actions by treating them as realities rather than possibilities.

Maintain and Add to Your Motivation

Everyone is highly motivated right before and after weight loss surgery. You are excited for your lifestyle change and determined to make it work. These are some of the reasons or motivations you need to stay on track early in your weight loss journey.

- Substantial weight loss.
- Preventing side effects and complications.
- A strong need to feel in control of your eating and your life.
- Desire to prevent a health condition or confront one that your obesity has caused.
- A longing to feel "normal" and fit into movie theater, restaurant, and airplane seats.
- The knowledge that you must get healthy or risk not being there for your family.

These reasons can inspire you to stay on course for a while. Then, the weeks after your weight loss surgery turn into months, and then into years. You may need to work harder to stay motivated. These possible sources of inspiration can emerge and stay with you as you progress in your weight loss journey.

- Having more energy as you lose more weight and get into better shape.
- Keeping up with friends and family in all kinds of activities.
- Shopping for and wearing smaller clothing sizes.
- Taking fewer medications.
- Feeling more comfortable in your own body.
- Feeling proud, not embarrassed, to be out in public.
- Training for a 5k road race, an exciting hike or a kayaking trip.

You should constantly be on the lookout for new sources of inspiration. Every weight loss milestone and non-scale victory should provide momentum for your good decisions. Each slip-up can be a reminder of why you are working hard.

Patience Is a Virtue ... and a Necessity

Weight loss takes time, even after weight loss surgery. A loss of 1 to 5 pounds per week is possible, but even with a good diet, getting to your goal weight can take years. You will have setbacks along the way. Some weeks you will not lose any weight. You might even gain a pound or two. Even when weight loss is steady, it can seem painfully slow.

Prepare yourself for slow weight loss, and for plateaus and setbacks. Do not try to speed your weight loss beyond what your surgeon and dietitian recommend. If you do, you risk developing complications, getting discouraged, and becoming malnourished.

Weight loss surgery requires patience for additional reasons. You can drive yourself crazy if you let yourself get frustrated by things that are out of your control.

- You may not be able to tolerate certain foods that you used to love, that you thought you would be able to tolerate by now, or that you could tolerate last week.

- You might be at a restaurant or a friend's house for a special dinner, take one or two bites, and suddenly find yourself too full or nauseated to eat another bite for the rest of the evening.
- If you are a lap-band patient, finding your "Green Zone" may take several months and several trips to the surgeon. The effort is worthwhile!
- You might have side effects or complications. To stay healthy, you need to find out their causes or wait until they go away rather than ignore them and try to lose weight faster.
- People can give you advice and opinions you did not ask for or do not agree with. Being patient with them instead of annoyed wastes less energy and increases your confidence and your ability to succeed.

Setting Goals and Celebrating Scale and Non-Scale Victories

Goals are important to weight loss and a healthy lifestyle. They let you measure your progress. Good goals are worth working hard for each day, and celebrating their achievement lets you recognize the value of your efforts.

Some of your goals are based on what the scale says. Sample time-based goals might be to lose 10 pounds this month or 80 pounds in the first year after surgery. Other goals can be based on milestones. These might include losing your first 50 or 100 pounds, getting under 300 pounds, or hitting your high school weight.

Not all of your goals should be related to weight, because you cannot really control the scale. Goals can be related to body measurements, participation in activities, and your own behaviors. These are some examples. Notice that even though they are not based on your weight, these goals are specific enough that you can tell when you achieve them.

- Fit into a size 12.
- Lose 4 inches around your waist.
- Take an aerobics class at the gym.
- Fit into a movie theater seat.
- Attend at least three bariatric support group meetings per month.

Goals should be challenging but realistic. A goal that is slightly difficult encourages you to work harder to reach it. These are some realistic goals and explanations of why they are realistic.

- *Lose an average of 1 to 2 pounds per week for the first six months after surgery.* This is weight loss that is achievable but requires a strict diet. Stating your goal as an *average* instead of a certain amount every single week allows for plateaus and uneven weight loss.
- *Work out four days this week.* This goal requires planning and dedication, but it also allows flexibility for the days when you do not have time to exercise.
- *Eat a serving of protein with each meal and snack today.* This goal requires planning and discipline, but it is a short-term goal, so you can have the focus needed to achieve it.
- *Order only a kid-sized hamburger and eat only the patty when you are forced to go to hamburger restaurants.* The challenge is to limit calories and avoid the hamburger bun, fried foods and sugars, but the goal recognizes that you cannot always avoid fast food restaurants.

A goal that is unrealistic sets you up for failure. If a goal is too hard, you might quit trying to achieve it, or be discouraged when you do not achieve it. These are some examples of unrealistic goals with explanations of why they are unrealistic.

- *Lose 5 pounds each week for the first two months after surgery.* Some weight loss surgery patients can achieve this weight loss, but losing this much weight consistently is unlikely. You might have post-surgery complications and need to focus on getting healthy before losing weight. Lap-band patients will not even get fills for several weeks after surgery. A more realistic goal is to follow your diet as well as possible in these two months to avoid complications, which will set you up for better weight loss later.
- *Wear a size 14 by Christmas.* Because you cannot predict exactly how fast you will lose weight, and you do not know which areas of your body will shrink fastest, you do not know how long it will take for your body to fit into a size 14.
- *Lose 10 pounds on my two-week vacation.* You may be eating different foods and have a different exercise schedule when you are on vacation. A more realistic goal is to maintain your weight loss while eating healthy foods and small portions.
- *Do not go to a restaurant until I lose 100 pounds.* Work and social obligations can force you to go to a restaurant. A better goal is to eat healthy food whenever you go out to eat.

Congratulate yourself out loud when you reach a goal. Brag about your accomplishment to your significant other or your other supporters. If you worked especially hard to achieve that goal, give yourself a treat, such as a new pair of walking shoes, an attractive new plate to use for your small meals, or maybe a manicure. Then set some new goals and keep working hard!

Non-scale victories (NSVs) are off-the-scale "wins." They may not be predetermined goals, but they can help you stay motivated. Recognizing them can take effort at first, but becomes easier and more rewarding with practice. These are some sample NSVs.

- You lose so much weight that your cousin does not recognize you when he flies in for your annual family reunion.
- Your daughter can sit on your lap because you now *have* a lap.
- You can bend over and tie your shoes.
- For the first time, you offer to go with your son or daughter to the school's mother-son or father-daughter dance.
- You go to a pro basketball game with your friends and only later realize that you did not even stop to look at the concessions.
- Your mother-in-law, who always has a derogatory comment about your appearance, only mutters something about your unnatural weight loss and funny eating habits.
- Your family vacation involved you *doing* something rather than *watching*.
- A stranger who does not know that you used to be obese compliments you on your appearance.
- You see your reflection in a store window and the first thing that comes to mind is "That person is pretty attractive!"

Fix Your Head

Experienced weight loss surgery patients know that your head largely determines your success. Some patients even describe the physical part of the weight loss journey as the easy part; you "only" need to eat right and exercise regularly. Many patients will tell you that the mental challenges are more difficult to overcome.

The sheer length of the journey is challenging. Your journey is not over with surgery, or within a few months, or when you hit goal weight. You need to follow your weight loss surgery diet, take your vitamins and mineral supplements and eat slowly for life. This can be discouraging if you feel like you will never be allowed to eat anything "good" again. Furthermore, the thought of being forced to do *anything* for the rest of your life is scary.

Focus on what you *can* do, not on what you *cannot* or *must* do. Simple changes in the way you phrase your thoughts can have real effects; just replace the negative thought with a positive thought about the same topic.

- "I can make myself a **chocolate protein shake** when I get to work this morning" instead of "I can't have my morning latté from Starbucks."
- "Now that I have more energy, I get to spend the afternoon at the mall with my friends," instead of "I can't go to the food court for a Cinnabon."
- "I get to listen to some of my favorite music in peace tomorrow," instead of "I have to go for a walk by myself tomorrow."
- "I get to play with my son and his friends at the park," instead of "I have to spend a whole afternoon with some kids, and I don't even get to have pizza with them."

You may have deep-rooted insecurities that contributed to your weight gain, grew during your years of being obese, and stuck around even through surgery. Recognizing and getting help for insecurities will help you gain self-confidence. When you are confident, you perform better at work and home, and are better able to stick to your weight loss plan.

Depression may be surprising if you are losing weight and your health is improving, but it is a common possibility after weight loss surgery. Many factors can contribute to depression.

- Surgery changes your entire life, including eating habits, daily activity, and personal relationships. These changes can be overwhelming even if they are generally positive.
- You might have some unaddressed emotions that you used to suppress by overeating, and now you need to face these full-on.
- You might be feeling guilty because you think you "should" feel happy but you don't.

Additional circumstances and feelings can also prevent you from feeling as proud and confident as you should feel.

- Anxiety over facing new situations and opportunities, such as ordering at a restaurant or buying a fitted suit for the first time after weight loss surgery.
- Concern over your appearance and excess skin that remains after losing weight.
- Conflicted or changing relationships
- Disappointment with your progress, especially if you have unrealistic expectations or goals, or if setbacks or complications occur that are out of your control and delay your progress.

Seek help if your negative feelings interfere with your daily life, make you feel hopeless, or outweigh the positive feelings. These feelings are common among weight loss surgery patients, and they can usually be well managed. That is why bariatric Centers of Excellence are required to be in contact with a mental health provider or psychiatrist, and they offer support group meetings and follow-up care.

You and the World

Life after weight loss surgery is easier if the people around you are supportive, positive, and caring. Most will be, and they should be part of your support system. Some people, though, will not be supportive. They may in many ways undermine you—intentionally or unintentionally.

- People might question you about your weight loss surgery until you feel like you're under a microscope or being grilled about a crime.
- They may tell you that weight loss surgery is cheating, dangerous, and/or ineffective.
- They may tell you "horror stories" they've heard about weight loss surgery.
- They may tell you "better" ways to eat and exercise, even if they do not know the first thing about weight loss surgery or your specific procedure.

One of the biggest problems that many weight loss surgery patients face is when someone else pressures them to go off their diets. This can range from unintentional and gentle suggestions to intentional and more forceful pressure.

- "Have some crackers and cheese while we chat. Just a bite won't hurt you!"
- "You eat like a bird. You must be malnourished by now!"
- "I made your favorite chocolate chip cookies; why don't you try one now while they're fresh?"
- "I spent all day making the fried chicken and biscuits that you love, and now you won't even eat them?"
- "I know you're on a diet, but you can diet any day. Let's go grab a couple of burgers and some fries."
- "Are you still measuring every bite? How silly and boring!"
- "You act like you think you're too good for the rest of us. You won't even eat our food."

The pressure does not have to be verbal. It can include:

- Keeping trigger foods in the kitchen even after you asked for them not to be.
- Intentionally or unintentionally "forgetting" what you can't eat and then serving it at a meal anyway.
- Arranging for get-togethers at restaurants you have specifically asked to avoid, even when you have suggested other suitable restaurants.
- Pointing it out whenever you eat something different than everyone else at the table.
- Refusing to serve a dish that you *can* eat when you are their guest.

Do not let other people drag you down.

- Be confident in yourself so that you can ignore negative people or words or actions.
- Grow thick skin. Insults, put-downs, and doubts are almost a certainty, but you do not have to listen to them. Mean people are not worth your energy.
- Anticipate what people can say or do to undermine your efforts, and prepare your reaction. The table below shows some examples.
- Avoid negative people as much as possible.
- Steer the conversation away from yourself and your weight.

Figure 22 – Common challenging questions – and polite responses

If they say…	…try answering:
You're too skinny already.	Thanks. My doctor is quite pleased with my progress and wants me to continue with my diet.
Come on. Just a bite won't hurt you.	It might. I've had a serious medical procedure that really limits what I can eat.
The holidays come around only once a year. Live a little!	I love the holiday season! I'm satisfied this year to be healthier and better able to appreciate family and friends. If I have some of that Christmas fudge, I might get sick and need to miss some of the fun our family has planned for this year.
You're no fun anymore. You say "no" to everything!	I'm sorry you feel that way. The way I feel is that I say "no" to many foods, but I am able to participate in more activities and enjoy my time with you more.
Don't you love me any more? I made your favorite chicken pot pie!	I love you very much and appreciate your taking the time to make it for me. Unfortunately, I can't eat that. I have had a medical procedure that may cause me to get sick if I eat it.
Why bother trying? You haven't lost any weight, so why are you depriving yourself?	Thanks for your concern. I'm still following my physician's instructions, and am feeling better with my new lifestyle.
You have failed at everything else. Why would you succeed at this?	I can't tell you for sure how this will turn out, but I am trying my best every day.
The gang is going out for Mexican food and a few beers. Are you coming, or are you going to be a spoilsport again?	Thanks – I'd love to join you! I'll bring my own snacks just in case the menu doesn't have anything for me.
Why aren't you eating? Don't you like the food?	Yes, the food is wonderful, thank you! I am full and can't eat another bite.
Here's your slice of John's birthday cake. I know you don't eat cake any more, but I know you want to let him know that you wish him a happy birthday!	Thank you, but I do not want to eat cake. This has been a very nice birthday dinner, and I am grateful that we have all been able to share this time and wish John a happy birthday.
You got weight loss surgery, so you don't have to diet.	Thanks, but my weight loss surgery will work only if I stick to my food plan. Otherwise I might get sick.
I just got off work and need a break! Do you want to come to dinner with me?	Yes, I'd love to, if you're willing to go to one of the restaurants that has food I can eat! Can you just give me 45 minutes so I can get in my workout first?
I never get to see you because you're too busy exercising and preparing your food now.	I'm sorry that's how you feel, but I appreciate your telling me. Because I'm so dedicated to my health right now, how would you feel about coming with me to the gym or for a walk? It would be great to have a chance to catch up with you!

For some weight loss surgery patients, all household members are willing to get rid of trouble foods such as ice cream, potato chips, and fish sticks. Most weight loss surgery patients are not so lucky, and one or more members of your household, especially children, are likely to feel like you are changing your dietary habits but they have the right to eat whatever they want. This can make your life a lot harder, but a reasonable compromise is often possible.

- If you or your spouse makes more of an off-limits food than is needed, freeze the extras immediately so you are not tempted to eat the leftovers.

- Plan your own treats. If you know your children and husband will be having apple pie after dinner, make yourself **stewed apples with cinnamon** to eat at the same time.
- Hide the goodies. If your children cannot live without cheese sandwich crackers, ask your spouse or oldest child to hide them and put one package in the children's lunches each day.
- Limit fast food at home. Ask your family members to finish their fast food meals before coming back home, or at least to buy only what they know they will eat so there are no leftovers for you to eat.
- Four days a week, pack your children a healthy lunch with the foods you keep at home. Let them choose one day each week when they will eat the school-provided lunch. Or pack a healthy lunch every day and then on Fridays, give them some money to buy a treat at school.

"You're Cheating!"

How many people have told you directly or indirectly that they think weight loss surgery is cheating? Many people think it is "the easy way out" because they think the pounds magically disappear after surgery. Some people are rude enough to accuse you of "cheating" to get skinny. These people are uninformed and disrespectful, and they are overstepping personal boundaries. How should you respond?

If you value their respect and think they will listen, you can gently explain how weight loss surgery works. Describe your procedure in as much or as little detail as you want, and let them know that you must now follow a medically-advised diet that will last for years.

You are not obligated to defend or explain your personal decisions to anyone, and that includes decisions on weight loss surgery. You might not want to explain your position, or you might not think that the person accusing you of "cheating" will listen to your explanation. You have every right to ignore them. Walk away or smile and change the subject. Don't bother getting angry; these people are not worth your energy.

Action is absolutely the best response to accusations that you're cheating. Keep up your hard work. Eat right and exercise day after day, month after month. Your accuser will see your dedication. If they don't, just focus on the goal. In a couple of years when you're at goal weight and proud of your looks, you won't care whether people think you "cheated" to get there. They probably won't remember anyway. Who knows, maybe they'll be chasing the latest diet fad and be jealous of your hard-earned success!

People and Relationships: Spouses, Children, Parents, Friends and Acquaintances

After weight loss surgery your attitudes, diet, health, appearance, and abilities change. With so many changes, your relationships can change, too. Often you can strengthen relationships, though it may take some effort.

Your spouse or partner may be your biggest supporter from the start. He or she can be ecstatic at your decision to get healthy and excited to have a partner who is more active and self-confident. To show support, your spouse might help you research the surgery, eat the same foods as you, and praise you for your hard work. Your relationship can grow stronger through the tough times, and become even stronger as you are able to do more things together as you lose weight.

On the other hand, your spouse may seem hostile toward surgery, or you may find your relationship feeling weaker after surgery. Try to see the situation from your spouse's perspective. Your partner may:

- be concerned that surgery is risky and not the answer to your obesity.
- be afraid that your new attitudes and lifestyle will change the balance in your relationship.
- feel jealous because you are spending more time preparing your meals and exercising, and less time together.
- feel burdened from "picking up the slack" if they have to temporarily do more of the household chores when you do not have as much time to do them.
- unintentionally be bad-tempered as a response to your higher stress levels.
- worry that your weight loss will increase your ability to earn money and reduce your dependence.
- worry that you will be less attracted to him or her as you lose weight.

Around half of all marriages end in divorce, and yours might not be strong enough to withstand your weight loss surgery. Challenges, though, can make strong marriages even stronger. Keep your spouse close to you with these strategies:

- Lean on him or her by clearly asking for what you need, whether that is silent support, help with meals, or learning more about your surgery to gain understanding.
- Constantly reassure that you still love your spouse, and always will, no matter what your weight.
- Find ways to spend more time together. Can you exercise together a few times a week, prepare your meals together, or set aside a weekly date night?

Depending on their ages, personalities and relationships with you, your children can be very supportive, absolutely against, or just neutral about your weight loss surgery. Children may demand to know why you do not eat what they eat or why you watch television only when you are on the treadmill or why sometimes you get sick after eating. Reassure your children and tell them the truth in terms they can understand. You may need to develop some guidelines about which foods they can have in the house, considering both your own needs and their desires. Your relationships with your children can be stronger than ever as you lose weight and have more energy to spend time with them.

In almost all cases, parents provide unconditional love and want nothing more than to see you be happy. Often one or both parents will be your reliable supporters during your weight loss journey. They can:

- be untiring cheerleaders.
- comfort and console you, just as they did when you were young, whenever you do not feel well or when you doubt yourself.
- check on you by phone, email, or in person.
- learn about your weight loss surgery and diet to understand what you are going through.

Despite your parents' love for you, they may not immediately be your biggest supporters. They can be against your surgery and weight loss journey because they think it is too risky. They may be afraid you will not lose weight and will become upset over this failure. They can even undermine your efforts with nasty comments because they feel guilty; they feel responsible that you are obese and struggling at all, and it seems easier to deny the situation.

Try not to get offended or discouraged. Let your parents in as much as they are willing, from explaining the surgical procedure and your diet, to asking them to help out with things like child care. Parents can be slow to change their minds, but can become supportive when they see it is working. There is no point in holding a grudge. Welcome your parents into your world when they are ready, and you might find that you develop the strongest relationship that you have ever had with your parents.

Friendships can also change after your weight loss surgery. True friends stick by your side no matter what, and you may be surprised to find who is supportive and who is not. Even if they are unsure that surgery was a wise decision, good friends will support you as soon as you make the decision. Your friendship can benefit as you become more energetic and healthier, so you can be a better buddy for all kinds of fun activities—and people who love you will be pleased that your health is improving.

Unfortunately, some friendships will not survive your weight loss journey. Some of your "friends" may feel threatened by your weight loss. Like a jealous spouse, they may fear that their "fat friend" will no longer depend on them for companionship, and that your needs will no longer take a back seat to their desires. As difficult as it is, let your hurtful friends go and keep the true friends. As the saying goes, "with friends like this, who needs enemies?" The good news is that as you lose weight and gain confidence, making new friends will become easier.

As you continue your healthy lifestyle and see each aspect of your life from a new perspective, take a careful look at your friends and their behaviors. We tend to keep similar diet and exercise habits as our social group does. If the friends and relatives you spend most of your time with tend to eat junk food and watch television, you probably will too. If they are health-conscious and active people, you probably will be too.

You do not have to leave your friends if they have unhealthy habits, but you should be aware of them and make a conscious effort to counteract them. Ask if you can meet for coffee instead of fast food, or go for a walk around the mall instead of a movie. Try to build a relationship around something other than food. If that is impossible, you may become distant from your former eating buddies. Preserve whatever parts of the friendship that you can, but be open to making new friends with more of your new interests.

Back to the Basics

Sooner or later, your weight loss will hit a hurdle, and more likely, you will encounter several hurdles. Your weight may plateau when you are trying to lose weight. When you are at your goal weight, you may start to re-gain weight. This is frustrating, scary, infuriating, and seemingly unfair. It's also normal and surmountable!

Don't panic when your weight starts to feel out of control. Instead, take a step back and look carefully at the situation. Ask yourself some basic questions. Have I been:

- ☐ so stressed or distracted recently that I have not been monitoring my diet?
- ☐ planning my food ahead of time so I always know what I am going to eat?
- ☐ ending each meal when I am full?
- ☐ getting enough protein, fluids, and other nutrients?
- ☐ choosing nutritious foods and avoiding high-calorie foods and beverages?
- ☐ logging *all* of my food?
- ☐ measuring *everything* that goes into my mouth?
- ☐ exercising as much as I should?
- ☐ staying in the green zone (lap-band patients)?

If you answer all these questions *honestly*, you will probably gain some insight into why the numbers on the scale are not what you expected. If it doesn't seem clear to you, you should make an appointment with your surgeon or nutritionist. Together you can figure out strategies to get your weight loss back on track or stop gaining weight back. They can also make sure that you don't have a health problem interfering with your weight loss.

How to Be Your Own Biggest Supporter

You are the person who experiences every second of your weight loss journey, bears the discomfort of surgery, and decides about every bite that goes into your mouth. *You* are the most substantial part of your support system.

You must stay motivated to succeed. If your weight plateaus, or if you start to regain weight because you no longer feel motivated, you can take steps to gain back your drive to succeed. List your reasons for having weight loss surgery and losing weight. They may include:

- ☐ preventing or managing health conditions such as diabetes, high cholesterol or blood pressure, or arthritis
- ☐ feeling more energetic
- ☐ looking better
- ☐ being around for your family for many more years
- ☐ enjoying a full life with normal activities
- ☐ wearing nicer clothes

Other reasons for sticking to your diet can be as simple as preventing side effects such as nausea, diarrhea, and heartburn, and feeling proud of yourself for making good decisions.

For inspiration, write your reasons for having the surgery and eating right in a single list or on post-its or blank stickers. Post your reasons where you can see them often. Display them on the refrigerator, in your car, in your wallet, and on your computer. Include some encouraging messages, your goals, and helpful reminders too. Be creative with your self-motivation!

- Stick "before" photos on your household mirrors so when you look at yourself now, you can see how far you have come.
- Hang your pre-surgery jeans or a t-shirt at the front of your closet to remind you that the journey is worthwhile.
- Pick a goal article of clothing, such as an old high school outfit or a cute outfit you will fit into at your goal weight, and put it at the front of your closet or on the back of the bathroom door.
- Set a goal date for an activity, such as a family hike or surfing lessons, that you could not do when you were at your starting weight. Count down to that date.

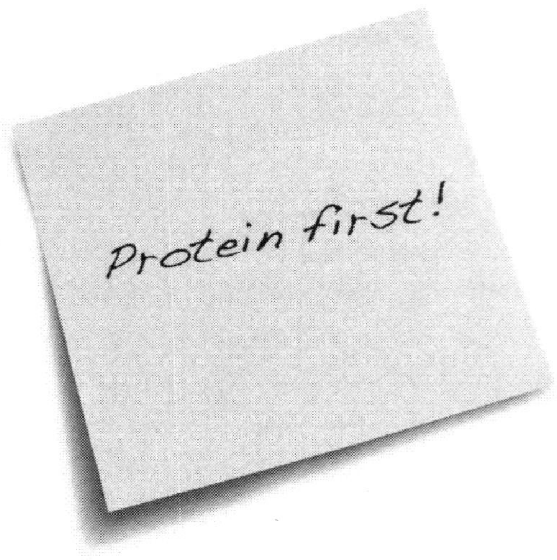

Post notes to yourself around your home and workplace, with little reminders and milestones.

- You've come so far!
- 100 pounds down!
- Protein first!
- Do it for your family!
- Skinny jeans!
- Use a photo on your mirror or a note on the calendar ("62 days till the boardwalk!")

These tips can help you become an even more effective self-supporter:

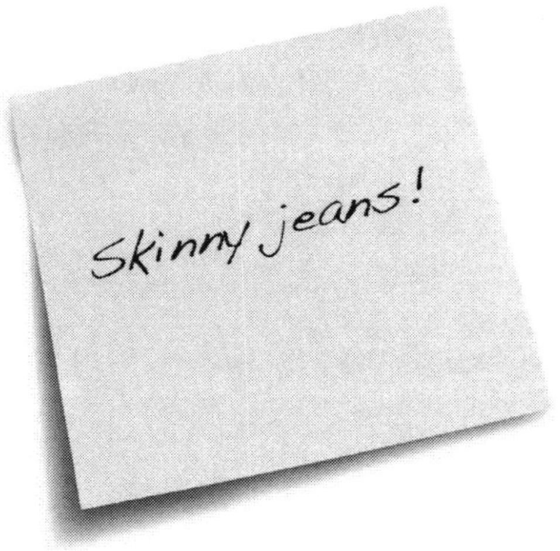

- Take away the doubt by practicing your responses ahead of time: "No, thank you," "No, I can't eat that any more," "No, I'm not hungry right now" can be automatic answers when someone offers you food that is not on your plan.
- Recognize and avoid trigger foods.
- Be positive and be a problem-solver. Forgive yourself when you slip up. Figure out *why* you slipped up, and how you will respond to the same situation in the future.
- Admit it when you need help, and reach out to your support system. Making specific requests can be the best way to make sure you get what you need, and it keeps the people who support you feeling useful.

Figure out which situations lead to negative self-talk or destructive actions. A log can help, as in the table below. Fill in some of your own examples.

Figure 23 – Recognizing and managing problem situations

Situation	Thoughts and Feelings	Result/Actions	Plan for Next Time
My mother-in-law said she can't understand how someone could have weight surgery and still look like I do. Then she served macaroni and cheese for dinner and ice cream for dessert, and had no healthy options for me.	I felt so ashamed. I felt like maybe surgery had been a waste of time and I'm a failure, so there's no point in trying to stick to my diet.	I did not answer her, but I lost control. I ate too much macaroni and cheese, and then ate ice cream too. I felt so bad that I skipped the walk that I had planned for that evening.	Stay proud and calm. I will bring my own dinner because it is my body. She can choose whether to offer something I can eat, but I can choose what to eat. I will focus on getting through the meal, and I will take out my anger during my evening walk.

Reexamine Your Support System

Before surgery, you built your support system to help you succeed. A good support system provides—as needed—encouragement, comfort, information, and reminders to stay on track. The network might include health care team members such as your physician, surgeon and nutritionist, along with family members, online and offline friends, acquaintances from work, religious organizations or clubs, and bariatric surgery support groups.

If you are straying off track, take a look at your support system. Is it still working for you? Have your needs changed? Consider the possibilities and solutions in the table below. You may need to adjust your support system if these or similar observations are true for you.

Figure 24 – Adjusting your support system to match your changing needs

Sample Shift in Your Needs	Sample Adjustment in Your Support System
You need more tough love to stay on track.	Ask your family members to not only encourage you, but also act as your conscience and gently mention unhealthy behaviors on your part.
You need less medical advice about complications and allowed diet foods, and more advice about recipes and adjusting to your new body, and more "been there, done that" advice.	Focus less on phoning your doctor's office for this and more on making connections with other WLS patients through support groups and online forums.
You've noticed some of your former supporters are no longer so supportive.	Either stay away from them or refrain from discussing your new lifestyle with them. They will just drag you down.
You have become more confident sharing your weight loss surgery story with others.	Include more people such as trusted work colleagues in your support system.
The daily grind of your weight loss journey is wearing you down.	Find other people who are in it for the long haul. They may be other WLS patients or just people with a lot of weight to lose who, like you, are following a strict diet program.

Figure 25 – Sample challenges and possible strategies

Sample Challenge	Possible Strategy
You have cravings for specific foods.	Have one bite of the food. If you cannot hold yourself to one bite, have an allowed substitute, such as diet hot cocoa for your chocolate craving. Or make a healthy substitute, such as high-protein **smashed cauliflower** instead of mashed potatoes.
It's not time to eat, but the kitchen is calling your name.	Distract yourself with a pre-determined activity. Try cleaning, blogging, talking on the phone, or taking a walk.
You are skipping your exercise routine.	Plan your workout the night before, arrange to meet an exercise buddy, and set a medium-term fitness goal to work toward.
You are a social eater; you have trouble sticking to your diet at parties and other occasions with food.	Eat your own high-protein snacks or drink water as a WLS-friendly alternative to party food.
Your friends like to meet for lunch.	Take your own high-protein, low-calorie meal or suggest that you meet for coffee or a walk instead of lunch.
You are an emotional eater.	Phone a friend, go for a walk, or go to the mall in the short-term. When the cravings pass, figure out why you were upset or stressed, what triggered the feelings, and how you can prevent them or manage them next time.

Practice Good Habits

Plateaus can happen when you lose focus and start to slip back into your old habits. To break through a plateau or prevent weight re-gain, continue work on your new lifestyle so your healthy actions replace bad habits. Go back to the basic strategies and rules you learned early in your weight loss journey.

- ✓ Chew slowly.
- ✓ Stop eating before you are full.
- ✓ Measure *everything* that goes into your mouth.
- ✓ Eat only at the table.
- ✓ Log your food and track your weight.
- ✓ Move, move, move.
- ✓ Eat your protein first.
- ✓ Don't drink your calories.

□

Exercise After Weight Loss Surgery

Weight loss surgery patients should exercise at least 30 minutes most days of the week, and more is better. Many patients start exercising almost immediately after surgery, while others wait because adjusting to the new diet is enough of a challenge at first. Whether you are a weight loss surgery newbie or veteran, the benefits of exercise are nearly unlimited.

- It burns calories to help you lose weight faster or maintain your weight loss. An online table or calculator can estimate how many calories you burn doing certain exercises.
- It improves your heart health because it lowers bad cholesterol, increases good cholesterol, and lowers blood pressure.
- It lowers your blood sugar if you have pre-diabetes or diabetes.
- It tones muscles, increases self-confidence, and makes you smarter, more productive, and happier.

You can meet your daily exercise recommendations and get these benefits from all kinds of exercises. To give you a few ideas, some are listed below. Exercise recommendations include at least 30 minutes on most days of the week, and more is better. You will get the benefits of exercise from these and other activities:

- Walking, hiking, and jogging
- Water aerobics, aqua jogging, and lap swimming
- Outdoors bicycling, spinning, and cycling on an upright or recumbent stationary bike.
- Playing basketball, volleyball, tennis, football, soccer, handball, raquetball, and golf (walk instead of using a cart)
- Dancing, aerobics, kickboxing, martial arts, and other group fitness classes
- Using a step machine (stair climber), elliptical trainer, or rowing machine at the gym or at home.
- Shoveling snow, weeding the garden, mowing the lawn, or raking leaves.

You already know you should exercise. If you are not yet a regular exerciser, it is either because you are having trouble getting started or because you have trouble staying committed to your program.

How Do I Start Exercising?

You can get started exercising as soon as you have your doctor's approval, at any point after weight loss surgery. You can be at any weight and fitness level, with any exercise experience (or no experience). Ask your doctor if you have any restrictions related to your surgery or health conditions. Then get started! These are some suggestions for beginners.

- Start with just a few minutes of very light exercise; walking up and down the driveway, walking in a shallow pool, pedaling slowly on a recumbent stationary bicycle, or just stretching exercises.
- Take advantage of any programs offered by your healthcare plan, e.g. appointments with a physical therapist.
- Ask an experienced friend for help.

- Grab a friend who wants to start exercising and learn the ropes together.
- Follow or modify our plan for beginners to get you from 0 to 30 minutes.

You do not need much equipment to start most exercise programs. A comfortable pair of walking or cross-training shoes, a T-shirt and a pair of sweatpants or shorts is adequate for most activities. You might want a water bottle and a towel. Other equipment may include a swimsuit if you are planning to be in the pool, and any needed equipment for sports such as a tennis.

Figure 26 – Four-week exercise start-up

Beginning plan to go from 0 to 30 minutes in four weeks. With your doctor's approval, you can follow this plan to work up to 30 minutes of walking in just a few short weeks. Start each workout slowly to let your heart rate increase gradually. Feel free to take a little longer to get through the plan; you can repeat each week one or more times. Feel free to modify the plan to suit your schedule.

	MON.	TUE.	WED.	THU.	FRI.	SAT.	SUN.
Week 1	5 minutes of slow walking.	Day off	5 minutes of slow walking.	10 minutes of walking.	5 minutes of cycling	Day off.	10 minutes walking.
Week 2	10 minutes of walking.	Day off.	5 minutes of walking plus 5 minutes of cycling.	10 minutes of walking.	15 minutes of walking	Day off	15 minutes of walking
Week 3	10 minutes of cycling plus 10 minutes of walking	15 minutes of walking plus 5 minutes of cycling	Day off	15 minutes of walking plus 5 minutes of cycling.	15 minutes of walking plus 10 minutes of cycling.	Day off	20 minutes of walking
Week 4	15 minutes of walking plus 10 minutes of cycling.	10 minutes of cycling plus 15 minutes of walking	Day off.	20 minutes of walking	15 minutes of walking plus 5 minutes of cycling	Day off.	30 minutes of walking

How Do I Keep Exercising?

Everyone who has started and quit exercise programs knows that keeping up with them is tough. Your record is perfect until an occasional workout slips by. Then you miss workouts regularly, two or three days in a row pass without exercise, and suddenly you realize you are no longer on your program.

Why is it so hard to stick to an exercise program? "I don't like exercising" is a common excuse, but it is almost never true. Try to figure out *what* you do not like about exercising, and avoid it or work around it. The table below lists some of common reasons people stop exercising, with suggestions for overcoming these obstacles.

Figure 27 – Common reasons to stop exercising, with solutions

Problem	Solutions
I don't have time.	Change your attitude. You do have time – you just have to figure out where it will come from. Give up watching television. Take a ten-minute walk on your break at work. Walk around the field, chase stray balls or do calisthenics while watching your child's soccer practice. Shoot hoops in the backyard with your children while talking about their school day. Use the stationary bike while you watch TV. See BP Book Time Management for more tips on using your time effectively.
I don't like exercise because it is too boring.	Listen to music, talk to an exercise buddy, watch a movie on television or work out in a park, hiking facility or shopping mall. Try multiple activities. You're much less likely to get bored if you walk two days a week, bike twice, dance once and play basketball once, than if you walk six days a week. Work toward a goal, such as running your first 5k or going rock climbing on your summer vacation. Then design your exercise program so that you'll be ready. Be creative. Figure XXX shows various activities to prevent boredom in and out of the gym.
I don't like exercise because it is too hard.	Try a slower warmup and only achieve your regular intensity after 5 or 10 minutes of slow walking or pedaling. Mix up your routine. Your body can get tired when you ask it to do the same thing day after day. Schedule some easy days, when you focus on enjoying your workout, and not on pushing yourself.
I am not making progress or seeing results.	Eating determines weight loss far more than exercise does. Exercise only burns a few calories compared to the amount you could eat if you are not careful. Try different activities. Let your muscles recover from one activity as you train them in another activity. Push yourself once or twice a week. Lift heavier weights, pedal faster for a few minutes or try some hills on the treadmill. Re-examine your goals. How are you measuring progress? You might not be getting faster, but is your resting heart rate coming down? Is your blood sugar under control? Are you able to exercise for longer?
I can't.	Yes, you can. You just have to find the right starting place for yourself. If all you can do is stand up and sit back down, do it as many times as you can. Work up from there. Increase the length of your walks. You may need to start by walking around the house. Then do it twice. Increase your laps around the house until you can make it down the driveway and back. Then walk down your street and back. Increase your length and eventually your speed. No matter what kind of shape you are in, you can do some sort of activity to improve your health.
I feel dumb.	You shouldn't. Most people are not judging you. Anybody who is judging you is not worth worrying about. The way to get over feeling "dumb" is to keep exercising so that you lose weight and get better at whatever activity you are doing.
The weather won't cooperate. It's too hot, cold, wet, windy or snowy.	Modify your workout. Hit the pool, beach or air-conditioned gym in the summer; pop in an exercise DVD at home in the winter. Conditions that are too dangerous to risk include icy streets, thunderstorms, tornado watches and other severe weather warnings. Take your workout inside. Change the time of day that you work out. Work out later in the day if you are waiting for the snow to be cleared from sidewalks. Work out early in the morning if the days are too hot. Work out at lunchtime if the mornings and evenings are too dark during the winter.

Figure 28 – Exercise should not be boring

These are some suggestions for activities that you can do to burn calories and get fit.

At the Gym
Cardio circuit: spend 3 to 5 minutes on the treadmill, elliptical, stationary bike, stair climber, or rowing machine. Then move to a different cardio machine. Switch machines every few minutes until you are done with your workout. *Strength training circuit*: After a few minutes of slow walking to warm up, perform a set of exercises for one minute. Then move to an exercise that works different muscles for a minute. Then try a third exercise that focuses on different muscles. Continue until you reach 10 different exercises. For a challenge, do the whole circuit twice so you get in a 20-minute workout. This circuit gives you cardio and strength training. (Example: 1 minute each of bicep curls, lunges, triceps extensions, squats, chest flies, dips, shoulder press, side lunges, calf raises and abdominal crunches.) *Mixed circuit:* Warm up, then mix up a cardio circuit and a strength training circuit. For the duration of your workout, alternate 3 minutes of cardio with 1 set of resistance exercises. *Group fitness classes*: spinning or cycling, aerobics, Zumba and boot camp are cardio classes. To help build strength, most gyms also offer pilates and classes that use dumbbells.
With Your Family
Romantic after-dinner walks with your partner. Age-appropriate activities with your children. Push your baby in a stroller to the store or walk while your child pedals a tricycle. Follow-the-leader or taking turns giving orders for activities, e.g. skipping, jumping, crawling or dancing. Hold dance-a-thons; take turns choosing the music and leading the steps. Shoot hoops, play catch, or kick around a soccer ball with your aspiring athlete. Do drills with your middle- or high-schooler who wants to play (or does play) on a team.
At Home
TV time: Record your favorite TV shows and watch them or your favorite movies while on the elliptical, stationary bike, or treadmill. You will be surprised at how good it feels to "earn" your TV time! *Exercise DVDs*: Get an assortment of DVDs so you get many different workouts. Possibilities include weight training, kickboxing, aerobics, and dancing. *Gardening*: pulling weeds, raking leaves, and digging dirt all burn calories. *Get moving* during commercial breaks by doing squats, knee raises, leg lifts, and arm swings. You can get in 20 minutes of activity just by moving during the commercial breaks during a 1-hour show. *Errands*: Walk or bike when you are not purchasing much. You can get a few items at the grocery store and go to the bank, post office, and library on foot or on a bike if they are near your home.

Make Friends at the Gym

Making exercise friends can be great for your long-term health and happiness. Being friends with other members of your gym can change your exercise program from a boring, short-term effort into a rewarding life-long program. Gym friends:

- Are motivating because they make the same long-term commitment for the same reasons: weight control and health.
- Hold you accountable so you come to the gym each day.
- Make the gym welcoming instead of cold and scary.

- Keep you company to make the time fly by. You can chat while you are next to each other on cardio machines and be partners for weightlifting.

Do not be afraid to try to make friends at the gym. Some members may be stronger, fitter, and more toned than you are now, but that does not make them snobs. They worked hard for that body and are still working hard, and that is the kind of body that you can have if you keep working hard. Try going to the gym at the same time each day so you can see who the regulars are, and try to make friends with them. Icebreakers can be awkward, but you'll get used to it. You can start a conversation by asking if they would like an exercise buddy. You can also tell them that you need motivation, or that you are a beginner so you would welcome advice on what to do at the gym. Some people might give you polite answers and move on, but others might be very open to conversation or even coaching. A few might tell you that they cannot talk right now. Do not take it personally; some people just prefer to work out alone.

Notes from Long-Time Exercisers

As a newcomer to exercise, you might wonder how some people can exercise regularly for years. Allowing yourself to think they have an advantage over you can discourage you from believing that you will be one of those people. This is some wisdom that nearly all long-time exercisers will tell you.

- It will always take effort. Just like you, they have trouble getting started and are sometimes tempted to quit.
- They give up other things just like you do when they go to the gym. Like you, they would be just as happy sleeping in, sitting on the couch watching television, or checking their email.
- It is a certainty in their days. They know that they will work out. Do not think about *whether* you will exercise, just know that you *will* exercise.
- Sometimes you have to make it a priority. This can mean going to bed earlier so you can get up earlier, taking a shower in a public locker room instead of at home, or packing a portable breakfast the night before instead of having a hot breakfast at home.
- Exercise is their personal time. They may like to work out alone, or with one or more buddies, in group classes or on sports teams, but they know that exercise time is their time to think, get fit, gear up for or wind down from the day, socialize and/or just be themselves.
- The rewards are worthwhile. They know they sleep better, perform better, and enjoy their days more with exercise. This motivation keeps them coming back day after day.
- They watch their diets carefully. They are as concerned about weight control as you are.

Log Your Workouts

Just as a food log helps keep your diet on track, an exercise log helps make your exercise program successful. Writing down your workout motivates you to do the workout. A log also makes it easier for you to see your progress. You can be as detailed as you want. Include the activity, how long you did it for, and any other details, including where you were, how you felt, and who was with you. The table below shows a sample weekly activity log. Write in your own sample activities beneath those listed.

Saturday	Sunday	Monday	Tuesday	Wednesday	Thursday	Friday
Weekly hike with Sarah. She pushes me hard, but we laugh so much. 2.2-mile Green Valley loop in 49 minutes. When we get better, we can park a little further away and get in a longer workout.	Katie and Jack had soccer practice at Marshall Park, so I walked/jogged around the field for 20 minutes. Then did some squats and lunges. Marsha's mom introduced herself to me and asked if she could join me. YES! I hope she will again.	Should have gotten up early but didn't. At least I made up for it a little bit at lunch. Walked with Paul and Jane to KFC – and didn't buy anything! Had my own lunch. 20 minutes of walking.	20 minutes of light dumbbells at home in early morning.	Family sports night! Katie picked basketball. First we did passing and dribbling drills, then scrimmaged a bit! Me and Katie against Joe and Jack. So much fun! 45 minutes.	Sore legs and back from b-ball yesterday. Easy walking 30 minutes at the gym.	Felt way better after yesterday's rest! 5 minutes easy cycling to warm up. Then awesome Tone-It class at the gym with my favorite instructor, Linda. 45 minutes.

Body Contouring and Skin Removal Surgery

You're starting to approach your goal weight and you feel great! You can be proud of yourself for sticking to your bariatric diet for this long, and for overcoming so many obstacles. You are enjoying your increased energy level, and you are rediscovering some of your body's long-forgotten curves and angles.

After losing a lot of weight, some weight loss surgery patients find that they have excess skin that is a problem. It can flap around when you run or do aerobics, dance, or other activities that require bouncing. It can get in the way of movement and make your daily activities uncomfortable. It can make you feel self-conscious and prevent you from being as proud as you should be about your weight loss and new looks. In some cases, sagging skin can threaten your health if it prevents you from washing yourself thoroughly or causes chafing and leads to infections.

Body contouring, skin removal surgery, or plastic surgery procedures can remove excess skin to let you move more freely. These procedures should be done only after you are at or near your goal weight, because you will develop more excess skin if you keep losing weight after skin removal surgery. These are some of the most common skin removal surgeries after losing a lot of weight:

- Brachioplasty, or arm lift, to remove excess skin under the arms
- Tummy tuck, or abdominoplasty, to remove excess belly fat and skin; it can also repair and firm weakened muscles
- Mastopexy, or breast lift, to make the breasts smaller and more comfortable during exercise and help improve posture
- Thigh lift to reduce sagging of the outer or inner thighs
- Body lift to help with sagging buttocks, abdomen, waist, hips, and outer thighs

The American Society of Plastic Surgeons (ASPS) recommends choosing an ASPS Member Surgeon who meets requirements for experience and ongoing education. Your pre-surgery appointment with the surgeon will be similar to your meeting with your bariatric surgeon. You might discuss why you want the surgery, potential risks, and pros and cons of the procedure. Your surgeon will take your body measurements, assess your health, and recommend treatment.

Body contouring surgery is usually an outpatient procedure. When you are discharged from the clinic, you will receive information on pain medications, keeping your surgery incisions clean, and avoiding activities that could split or compromise your incisions.

Should you get skin removal surgery? It can help you keep the weight off long-term if:

- it improves your motivation to stick to your diet.
- excess skin discourages you from exercising.
- excess skin makes you feel as though the surgery and your hard work are not worthwhile because you still *feel* overweight.

Body contouring surgery is a big decision, and you should consider both sides.

- If you gain weight back, you may have stretch marks.
- You may be disappointed if you go into the surgery with unrealistic expectations. If you do not look like a movie star with excess skin, you will not look like one after skin removal surgery.

- All surgeries have risks, such as infections, although the risks from body contouring surgery are smaller than for other surgeries.
- Surgery can be expensive. It is rarely covered by insurance because it is considered an elective surgery and not a medical necessity.

Restaurants After Weight Loss Surgery

Restaurant meals can be challenging after weight loss surgery. Portions are too big, and menu items are often high-calorie, starchy, and high-fat. You can have trouble finding the lean protein on your weight loss meal plan. Avoiding restaurants altogether may seem easiest, but it's not always an option. You will almost certainly find yourself at a restaurant at least occasionally with your family, friends, or work colleagues.

Although you need to be careful, you can eat at restaurants and still lose weight. Do your best to follow the same basic bariatric surgery diet guidelines that you follow with a home-prepared meal or snack.

Figure 29 – Diet guidelines and tips for restaurants

Guideline	Tips
Eat slowly.	Put your fork down after each bite, and chew thoroughly. Talk and listen to your companions to slow down your eating. This can also help you enjoy the entire experience more.
Eat protein first, then vegetables.	Skip the breadsticks, tortilla chips, and dinner rolls that come before the meal. Ask your server not to bring them, or at least place them out of reach. Do not order an appetizer; most are high-fat and high-calorie. If you must have an appetizer, choose one with lean protein: grilled shrimp or a raw vegetable plate. Be sure your main course has a source of lean protein; eat that first. Pick out the protein from the dish and eat it. Examples include chicken in wraps and veggie burger patties in sandwiches.
Avoid fluids within 30 minutes before or after a meal.	Do not order soup before your meal. Order soup only if you are not eating solid foods at the meal, and choose a broth-based soup, not a creamy soup. Drink some water a half hour before entering the restaurant. A half hour after you've eaten, drink some more water.
Choose low-calorie nutritious foods.	When possible, check the protein and calorie content of foods ahead of time or at the restaurant. Search for lean proteins, vegetables prepared without fat, and fresh fruits without sugar. Ask your server not to bring extra items, such as French fries, that are not on your diet.
Eat small meals.	Do not order oversized or double portions, even if they are "bargains." Order the smallest portion. Split your meal with your companion. Ask your server to bring a "to-go" box when your meal is served. Plan how much you eat before you start eating. Pack up the rest to take home for later. The estimates in BP Book Measuring Food can help you estimate portion sizes.

Planning ahead is always best. If you know where you are going ahead of time, you can usually look at the menu online. Check nutritional information if it is available. Pick out a high-protein option that is low-fat and low-calorie. Also look for steamed or grilled vegetables, with a green salad or fruit. You can call ahead to find out whether the restaurant is willing to serve you certain items, such as cottage cheese or baked unbreaded fish, that may not be listed on the menu.

If the restaurant's menu does not meet your needs, bring your own food. You can, for example, eat your own protein bar with a restaurant salad, or sprinkle your own protein powder on the restaurant's low-fat soup.

You will not always know ahead of time that you will be going to a restaurant or where you will be going. Do not panic! Do your best to pick out the best choices from the menu, aiming for a high-protein, low-sugar, low-fat meal. Certain words on menu items can alert you to good and bad bets.

Figure 30 – What to choose and what to avoid at restaurants

Look for or ask for:

- ✓ Steamed
- ✓ Grilled
- ✓ Baked
- ✓ Roasted
- ✓ Poached
- ✓ Boiled
- ✓ Marinated
- ✓ Fat-free
- ✓ High-fiber
- ✓ Fresh
- ✓ Diet
- ✓ Broiled
- ✓ Low-carb

Avoid:

- X Fried, deep-fried, sautéed, pan-seared: fried foods are not on your diet.
- X Crispy, frittered, or golden: other words to describe fried food
- X Battered, breaded, en croute or crusted: extra carbohydrates from bread crumbs or crust, with extra fat
- X Sticky, glazed (extra sugar)
- X Creamy
- X Stuffed
- X Sticky (likely sugary)
- X Au gratin, scalloped, smothered, carbonara: extra cheese, butter or cream
- X Confit: salted high-fat meat
- X White sauce, béchamel, roux, hollandaise, bearnaise: buttery sauces
- X Special sauce: usually high-fat
- X Bisque – cream soup
- X Tempura – breaded and fried

Your Server Can Help

Before ordering, ask your server about any item you are unsure about. For example, how is the Low-Fat Seasoned Chicken served? It may come on a bed of pasta, accompanied by breadsticks and served with soup as an appetizer. You cannot have the soup before you eat solid foods, because you must have at least 30 minutes between drinking fluids and eating solid foods. Plus, pasta and breadsticks are starchy and high-calorie. They may even cause a band blockage (lap-band patients) or dumping syndrome (gastric bypass patients). On the other hand, the Low-Fat Seasoned Chicken may come with steamed broccoli and fresh fruit. Your server can explain each menu item that you are interested in, and it's often possible to substitute a healthy and nutritious choice (steamed vegetables) for a not-so-healthy choice (fried potatoes).

In most restaurants where food is made-to-order, you can ask about substitutions. You might ask to substitute a side salad instead of a fatty appetizer, a lettuce wrap instead of bun, and broiled fish instead of fried. These substitutions are often free, but in some locations you may need to pay extra for them. These are some questions to consider asking your server:

- ☐ Do you have any dishes with grilled or baked chicken, fish, or shellfish?
- ☐ May I have steamed vegetables or fresh fruit or a side salad?
- ☐ Do you have any low-calorie options?
- ☐ May I have the sauce/dressing/gravy on the side?
- ☐ Could the cook make the dish without butter/oil/cream?
- ☐ Can you please not serve bread and butter (or chips and salsa, or breadsticks and oil)?
- ☐ How is the dish prepared?
- ☐ May I have it grilled or baked instead of fried?

- May I have steamed vegetables instead of rice?
- Could you please bring a to-go box when you bring the order?
- I don't see anything on the menu that I can eat. Could you please bring me some cottage cheese and plain canned tuna?
- May I please have my omelet made with egg whites instead of whole eggs?

Some restaurants may not appear to have anything you can eat, but they can probably find something that is in the kitchen and not on the menu. Most casual restaurants have many of the suggestions in the table below in their storeroom or pantry, if not on their menus. If you cannot find anything diet-friendly on the printed menu, try to build your own healthy meal by asking for a lean protein and a vegetable, fruit, or nutritious starch.

Figure 31 – Best bets at restaurants

Most restaurants have the lean proteins, dairy, vegetables, fruits and starches that you need! You can build your own meal by asking for these common foods.

Lean Protein	Vegetables and Fruits	Starches and Starchy Vegetables
Grilled chicken (often available on a salad or in a sandwich)	Side salad	Cold breakfast cereal (whole grain)
Fat-free cottage cheese	Steamed vegetables	Plain oatmeal or hot cereal, with pecans
Lean deli turkey breast or ham	Raw vegetables	Plain baked potato
Veggie burger	Grilled seasonal vegetables	Sweet potato (no butter)
Turkey burger	Garden salad	Corn on the cob (no butter) – but lap-band patients may not be able to tolerate corn.
Egg whites	Fruit cup	
Low-fat or fat-free yogurt	Whole apple, orange or banana	
Canned tuna	Applesauce	
	Apple slices	
	Grapes	
	Melon	

Fast Food—You Can't Avoid It!

After weight loss surgery, you avoid fast food as much as possible. It can be greasy, sugary, and starchy. You can be tempted to increase your portion sizes and add high-calorie sides and drinks to get more food for your money. Drive-throughs encourage you to buy food, whether you are hungry or not, and to eat it in the car instead of sitting at the table. In many ways, eating fast food is the opposite of what you should be doing on your weight loss surgery diet.

Despite your best intentions, you may find that avoiding fast food completely is unrealistic. Your children might beg for it, your co-workers might drag you to it at lunchtime, or you yourself might need to turn to it if you have not had time to prepare your meal.

You *can* choose a meal or snack that fits your meal plan. You just have to know how. Stick to your usual strategies of emphasizing lean proteins and vegetables, limiting starches, fats, and sugars, and keeping portion sizes small.

Suggestions for some of the most popular types of fast food and ethnic restaurants, including the ten largest chains in the United States.

Figure 32 – Tips for surviving fast food stops

Type of Food or Restaurant	Look for:	Tips/Skip
Hamburger (McDonald's, Wendy's, Burger King, Sonic, Jack in the Box, Hardee's, Carl's Jr.)	Small burger (don't eat the bun) Grilled chicken salad or sandwich (skip the bread) Oatmeal with pecans (skip the brown sugar) Yogurt parfait (skip the granola) Apple slices Egg white English muffin breakfast sandwich Snack wrap (use a fork and eat it out of the tortilla)	Double burgers Fries, onion rings and fried zucchini Value-sized portions Special sauce, cheese and mayonnaise Breakfast sandwiches on croissants and Biscuits Bacon Shakes and smoothies Fried chicken and fish Chicken nuggets and strips
Sandwich (Subway, Quizno's, Jimmy John's)	Salad with vegetables and grilled chicken, turkey breast, or ham Egg white sandwich on English muffin Low-carb "unwich" (without bread) or wrapped in lettuce Apple slices Low-fat yogurt Chili	Fatty meats Cheeses Tuna or seafood salad with mayonnaise Chips and cookies Dressings and mayonnaise Meatballs and steak
Mexican (Taco Bell, Chipotle, Qdoba)	Small chicken or steak taco without cheese Side of black beans "Naked" burrito or salad without cheese or chips and with salsa, grilled vegetables and grilled chicken or steak. Fajitas	"Supreme" Sour cream and cheese Tostadas, tortilla chips and nachos Burritos Fried chalupas, taquitos and chimichangas
Pizza (Pizza Hut, Domino's, Papa John's, Little Caesar's)	Chicken wings (remove the skin) Garden salad (light dressing on the side) ½ slice thin-crust pizza without cheese Extra vegetables, anchovies, ham or grilled chicken as toppings Marinara, pizza and BBQ dipping sauce	Thick and stuffed crust Sausage, pepperoni and bacon toppings Extra cheese Ranch, cheese, garlic, and honey mustard dipping sauce Breadsticks
Coffee Shops and Bakeries (Starbucks, Dunkin Donuts, Panera)	Plain hot decaffeinated coffee or tea Yogurt Salad (light dressing) with grilled chicken Oatmeal with fresh fruit ½ sandwich with vegetables and turkey breast on whole-grain bread Chicken noodle, vegetable, lentil or bean soup (if not eating solid foods) Low-carb/high-protein menu items	Doughnuts, pastries, cookies, cakes, scones, muffins Oversized bagels (your serving size is 1 oz. or ¼ of a typical bagel) Croissants Milk-based and sweetened coffee and fruit drinks
Chicken (Chick-Fil-A, KFC, Popeye's)	Grilled chicken Green beans Side salad (light dressing) Corn on the cob (no butter) Barbecue sauce, hot sauce	Fried or crispy or popcorn chicken Coleslaw Gravy, biscuits, pot pie Macaroni and cheese Dessert Ranch, honey mustard, and creamy dipping sauces

Figure 32 continued: Suggestions for some of the most popular types of fast food and ethnic restaurants, including the ten largest chains in the United States.

Type of Food or Restaurant	Look for:	Tips/Skip
Asian (Chinese, Korean, Thai, Vietnamese, Japanese restaurants)	Brown rice Steamed vegetables Chicken, shrimp, fish and tofu Small serving of sushi (be careful of sticky rice) Teriyaki chicken Soy sauce, oyster sauce, fish sauce Seaweed salad Steamed fish Lychee	Fried rice (or more than a bite of white rice) Chow mein Egg rolls or tempura Fried crispy noodles Breaded or crispy chicken or shrimp (e.g., Kung Pao chicken) Sweet and sour dishes Coconut-based dishes Red curry Fried bananas
Indian	Tandoori chicken Shish kebab Chicken or beef tikka Vegetable or lentil curry without a cream base	Cream curry Korma Samosas Pakora Saag paneer Ghee (clarified butter)

Never Give Up!

Do not give up, no matter how bad your options look. Throwing in the towel can lead to overeating and stretching your stomach pouch or gastric sleeve. Eating too much fat or sugar can cause dumping syndrome, especially in gastric bypass patients. Eating doughy bread and tough meat can cause lap-band complications. Regularly eating high-calorie food can derail your weight loss.

One big challenge is a restaurant that does not offer the foods you need. Another is when someone else does the ordering for you, so you have no say in the matter. Another challenge is going to a restaurant without previous warning, so you cannot check nutrition facts and menu options online. These strategies can improve the situation and help you stick to your diet.

Strategy 1: Be Picky.

You do not have to eat the entire meal as served. Instead, pick out the protein and other parts of the dish that your diet allows. For example, if you eat an entire a Big Mac, you'll get 550 calories, 29 grams of fat, and 46 grams of carbs. If you scrape off the sauce, throw away the bun and just eat the beef patty, cheese, lettuce, onions and pickle, you'll have 240 calories (less than half!), 4 grams of carbs (about one-eleventh!) and 18 grams of protein. If you have pepperoni pizza and just eat the cheese, pepperoni, and sauce, you will consume 140 calories and 6 grams of protein. Eat the fillings of sandwiches and burritos, pick out the chicken and vegetables from pasta, and eat the lettuce and eggs from salads but leave the croutons and fatty meats.

Strategy 2: Eat Less.

If you feel embarrassed picking through your food, just limit your portion size. A half slice of pepperoni pizza has 150 calories, 17 grams of carbohydrates, and 12 grams of protein. That's more carbohydrates than you need at a meal, but you can make up for it the rest of the day. Take small bites, chew slowly, and talk to your companions so that you do not feel tempted to eat more.

Strategy 3: Bring Your Own.

It's okay to bring your own protein bar and eat it when others are eating junk food. This strategy works at parties, work functions, and casual and fast-food restaurants.

Fast Food and Casual Restaurant Breakfasts

Traditional breakfast foods can be devastating to your diet with their calories, carbohydrates, starches, sugars, and saturated fat. They can cause dumping syndrome, blockages, nausea, and blood sugar swings. Avoid the following high-calorie, low-nutrient options:

- ☐ Starchy waffles, pancakes and French toast
- ☐ Sugary, fatty and starchy pastries and doughnuts
- ☐ Starchy and fatty croissants and biscuits
- ☐ Fatty sausages, bacon, and cheese
- ☐ Sugary syrup, jam, and jelly
- ☐ Fatty and starchy hash browns, potato hash, and potato pancakes

Instead, try the following:

- ☐ Oatmeal: skip the brown sugar topping and add your own protein powder
- ☐ ½ single-serving packet of peanut butter and one-third of a whole-wheat bagel
- ☐ Egg white omelet with salsa
- ☐ Fat-free or low-fat yogurt or cottage cheese with fresh whole fruit or fruit salad
- ☐ Breakfast sandwich on an English muffin: eat only half the muffin and top it with turkey bacon, ham, or egg whites.

Special Occasions

Life continues after weight loss surgery. So do social obligations, family gatherings, parties, and holidays. These events make life worth living, but many weight loss surgery patients fear them for good reason. First, most social events seem to center around food. Second, you may feel self-conscious about your weight loss surgery, especially if some people at the gathering do not know about it or respect your decision and diet.

Small Get-Togethers

When planning a small gathering, your friends or family members might automatically assume that you will be meeting for a meal. Suggest an alternative activity that allows you to enjoy each other's company but doesn't revolve around food. A nature walk or some window shopping in a mall or on a chic downtown street is ideal because you can burn some calories while you talk. Even sedentary activities such as watching a DVD movie or playing cards or a board game are healthier than centering your visit around a high-calorie meal that can stall weight loss or make you sick.

You can still salvage your diet even if your friends and family insist on meeting for a meal. If they want to go to a restaurant, try to persuade them to go to a restaurant where you are sure you can enjoy a high-protein, low-fat meal. Follow the tips in the restaurants section of this book to order smart and eat healthy food.

Your friends may want you to come over and enjoy their hospitality. Having a meal at the home of a friend or family member can lead to tricky situations, but your host will often be sympathetic to your needs. Ask what will be on the menu and explain your dietary needs when you are first invited over. Ask if you can bring a dish, and suggest one that's healthy and safe for you and delicious for others, too. One or two small changes or additions to the planned menu can change the meal from a diet disaster—and possibly a cause of complications for you—and a pleasant occasion with good company and a reasonably healthy meal. These ideas are easy for any host to implement.

- Serving a green salad with a low-fat dressing on the side
- Serving steamed or **roasted vegetables** instead of vegetable casseroles or vegetables with butter or cream sauce
- Grilling or baking the meat, chicken, or fish instead of serving it breaded
- If the menu is already set and the food on it sounds impossible for you to work with, politely ask your host if you can bring your own. Reassure him or her that this is your first choice, and you appreciate the opportunity to enjoy their company at their table while eating a meal that has your doctor's approval.

Another option for home gatherings is to bring a dish that the host or hostess can serve to everyone. This alternative can make you less self-conscious, because you will be eating the same food as everyone else, and it solves the problem of what you should bring for the host as a polite gift. Recommended options include deviled eggs, Greek yogurt dips, low-fat bean dip, Southwestern shrimp, four-bean salad, and cheesy spinach mushrooms—all of which can be found in the recipe section at the back of this book.

Sticking to Your Weight Loss Surgery Plan at Parties

Although you have less control over the menu, you can still have a good time and come out on top with your eating when attending catered events such as wedding receptions, work functions, and bar and bat mitzvahs. Always make a plan and have a backup plan in mind.

Think about what foods are likely to be served, and which you can and should not eat. The same rules apply at parties as at every other meal. Keep your portions small, focus on protein and vegetables, and eat slowly. These are some other tips for buffet-style events.

- ☐ Sit or stand far from the food table so you are not tempted to refill your plate.
- ☐ Use the smallest plate available.
- ☐ Look over the entire food table before serving yourself food. Decide what you will eat and how much, and then serve yourself.
- ☐ Do not return for seconds.
- ☐ Take small portions. Look at the section on measuring your food for info on eyeballing.
- ☐ If you are mingling with the other guests, hold a glass of water in your hand to keep yourself occupied so you don't eat.
- ☐ Concentrate on enjoying the company of the other guests. You'll have more fun at the party and eat less, too.
- ☐ When you have finished eating, remove your plate and enjoy a sugar-free mint.
- ☐ Don't drink alcohol. It is high-calorie and can make you less likely to resist high-calorie foods.

Figure 33 – Choosing foods at buffets

Choose lean proteins, vegetables and fruits	Avoid foods high in calories, fat, sugar and starch.
✓ Turkey breast, ham or other low-fat deli meat	X Egg rolls and crab Rangoon
✓ Shrimp cocktail	X Pepperoni, salami and other fatty Italian meats
✓ Chicken kabobs	X Dips – spinach, cheese, ranch, crab, artichoke
✓ Fresh-cut vegetables	X Fried foods (wings, shrimp, cheese sticks, jalapeño poppers)
✓ Salsa	X Chips, snack mixes
✓ Roasted vegetables	X Tarts, dough-wrapped appetizers (pigs in blankets, puff pastry appetizers)
✓ Fresh fruit – often served on cheese platters or as Fruit kebabs	X Mini pizzas, mini burgers (or just eat the patty if necessary), quesadillas, mini sandwiches
✓ Plain seafood	X Bread-based appetizers
✓ Limit nutritious, high-calorie foods to a small serving	X Cheese balls
✓ Cheese cubes	X Pasta
✓ Nuts or peanuts	
✓ Hummus	
✓ Olives	

Eating right is trickier when you are at an event with table service and a pre-determined menu, but you can still stay on track.

- ☐ The first chance you get, tell your server that you have dietary restrictions. Ask if you can have your salad with dressing on the side, and whether there are any other ways to make order your meal low-fat. Your server may be willing to bring you grilled or roasted chicken and steamed vegetables instead of the meal that everyone else is getting.

- Look at your plate carefully before starting each course. Decide exactly what and how much you will eat. Use your silverware to divide the food that you plan to eat from the food you do not plan to eat.
- Pick out the foods that are on your diet, and skip the rest. For example, you can eat your salad greens but leave the croutons untouched.
- Pass the bread basket out of reach.
- Place your napkin over your plate and push your plate away from you when you are done eating so you are not tempted to pick at the remaining food.
- Ask your table's server not to bring you dessert.

Is all of this too complicated for you? Fall back on your trusty can't-fail protein bar. You can eat it for a guilt-free meal or snack at any event, whether self-service or table service. Your dietary needs are just as important as anyone else's.

Sticking to Your Party Plan

Think about this scenario. You are looking forward to the annual party held at your company CEO's home. This year's party will be the first one since your weight loss surgery. You make your game plan and are confident you can stick to it—that is, you are confident until you knock on the front door and the CEO welcomes you with, "It is so nice to see you! May I offer you an appetizer?" All you see on the tray are mini quiches, crostini with bleu cheese, and puff pastry stuffed with bacon and cheese. You do not want to be rude, so you take a quiche and start nibbling it as the two of you talk. But then you're offered a second appetizer, and just to be polite, you accept the offer.

Five minutes into the party, you have already gone off your plan despite your best intentions. How can you prevent this from happening?

Think ahead. Before going to the party, try to predict what people might say or do so that you are not caught off-guard. This can keep you from feeling flustered or insulted, so you will be more likely to make wiser decisions at the party. Be prepared for:

- People who offer you forbidden foods and act insulted or disappointed if you refuse.
- People who make you feel self-conscious or defensive with comments about topics that are none of their business: your weight or your food choices.
- Tempting foods that appear from all directions at all times.
- Sudden fullness and the inability to eat another bite.

Rehearse your responses. Sooner or later, you may be tempted to go off your diet at a party when someone offers you food. So you don't end up eating extra calories, practice responses ahead of time in your head, in front of the mirror, or with your partner. They should roll off your tongue naturally.

- "No, thank you."
- "Thank you. I am full right now, but may try a bite later."
- "Thank you. I already enjoyed my appetizers, and I'm saving room for the main course."
- "Excuse me, but could you please bring me a plate without the rice pilaf?"

- "Oh! I have been having so much fun talking to the other guests that I haven't even had time to eat! I will help myself to some of that soon. It looks delicious!"
- "This spinach ravioli and cream sauce looks wonderful. Unfortunately, some recent health issues are keeping me from eating rich foods. I hope you don't mind if I can't eat with you right now."

Have an action plan. How will you prevent and overcome sticky situations? Design an action plan before the party so you know what to do when trouble threatens. These are some more suggestions to help you:

- Think before reacting. You can be caught off-guard by the mini egg rolls that you used to love, by a server setting a plate of beef wellington and scalloped potatoes in front of you, or by an offhand personal comment about your weight, your surgery, or your diet. Don't dive into the egg rolls, wolf down the high-fat beef and potatoes, or start eating mindlessly. Instead, continue on with your eating plan. Ignore the egg rolls; ask the server to bring you a healthier choice, or eat only the beef while leaving the puff pastry and potatoes on your plate. Definitely ignore the offensive comments.
- Repeat mantras to yourself. I can do this. I'm strong. I will eat only what I choose to eat. I am in control. Nobody can make me eat anything I do not want to eat. *Believe and act on your mantras.*
- When the party involves mingling, keep your water glass full and carry it around so your hands are too busy to hold a plate and fork.
- Delay your next helping of food. You can watch the clock to help pass the time without overeating. Mentally divide the party into smaller chunks. Tell yourself, for example, that you can wait until the current high-calorie course is cleared away or that you will refrain from eating and refill your water glass in 10 minutes. Tell yourself you will refrain from eating for at least another 15 minutes until you use the restroom, or that you will stop eating now and just enjoy a mint for 10 minutes. It is much easier to postpone eating for a few minutes at a time than to tell yourself that you will not eat at all for the next several hours!
- Be the life of the party. Talk to people at your table or anyone in the room, even if they are strangers, and you will find that you are less focused on food. Are you shy? Recruit your partner or a trusted friend to introduce you to people and start conversations. If talking doesn't come naturally to you, prepare some small talk you can use. Ask a neutral question and be ready to follow up on the answer or give your own opinion. Safe topics include:
    - The weather
    - Upcoming holiday or vacation plans
    - How the person you are talking to met the party's host
    - What the person's job is (or role in the company, if at a company function)
    - The delicious food, beautiful décor or view, or lively entertainment
    - The person's nice clothing, earrings, or hairstyle
- Get into the habit of automatically estimating food calories and converting them into minutes of exercise. That should motivate you to avoid the extra portion.

Figure 34 – The motivation to say "no" to extra foods at parties.
Estimates of exercise times are based on a 250-pound person.

Food Item	Calories (Approx.)	Exercise Needed to Burn It Off
Dinner roll with butter	300 calories	24 minutes of swimming laps
1 small spinach and cheese puff	70 calories	10 minutes of bicycling
1 cocktail frank with cheese	200 calories	30 minutes of slow walking
1 cup chicken fettucine alfredo	400 calories	30 minutes of hiking
1 handful of mixed nuts	400 calories	45 minutes of brisk walking
1 small slice of cheesecake with raspberry topping	300 calories	50 minutes of aerobics

Parties should be fun—and they can be fun! Parties are about people and celebrations. Dance, talk and laugh, and stay focused—you just might discover that you feel freer without food as a distraction.

The Holidays

"The holidays" would not be so difficult if they included only the actual holidays, such as Halloween, Thanksgiving, Christmas or Hanukah and New Year's. The reason they are so challenging for your diet is that "the holidays" are more like "the holiday season." The season includes:

- Halloween parties, trick-or-treating, and leftover candy
- Thanksgiving dinner *and* leftovers
- Holiday parties at work and at friends' houses
- Get-togethers with rarely seen friends and family revolving around food
- Edible holiday treats around the office and edible gifts
- Leftovers!

It seems as though food is *everywhere* from mid-October through early January, and choices are mostly high-calorie, high-sugar and/or high-fat—the opposite of the low-calorie, high-protein, nutritious foods you need to lose weight. The stress of the season can let old habits like emotional eating sneak back into your life. To make matters worse, exercising can be more difficult. You may have less time to fit in workouts if you are extra busy at work or with social obligations, and the start of winter can make exercising outdoors more difficult.

Poor eating for these months can cause weight gain. It can also lead to complications or side effects, especially if you are not far out from surgery. Sweets can cause dumping syndrome (roux-en-Y patients), sticky candies and stuffing can stick in the band (lap-band patients), and overeating can stretch your stomach pouch or sleeve, not to mention make you feel sick.

Weight gain and side effects can happen if you slip back into old habits, but they are preventable. To enjoy the holiday festivities without damaging your health or weight loss, first relax. Do not put too much pressure on yourself. The average person gains less than 2 pounds over the holidays. That's more than you want to gain, but it is far less than the 5 to 10 pounds that many people fear. Modifying your weight loss expectations can build confidence and help you hit your goals. Set your goals to lose weight a little more slowly or even to just maintain your weight during this period so you do not get frustrated and give up.

Prepare your defense by planning ahead. For example, if you know that the reception desk has your favorite chocolate truffles, avoid walking by the area as much as possible. If you need to go by the desk, carry papers so your hands are full and you cannot help yourself to truffles. Keep some sugar-free hot cocoa mix handy in case your chocolate craving gets too strong. A 3-piece serving of chocolate truffles has 210 calories and 15 grams of sugar, while a packet of diet hot cocoa mix has just 25 calories and 2 grams of sugar. These are some other ideas to stay on track during the holidays:

- Keep using a food journal to log everything, even junk food! You're less likely to sneak a Christmas cookie when you know that you have to write it down.
- Before you start each meal, figure out exactly what and how much you will eat. When you reach that point, use a strategy to end your meal. Leaving the table is best; if you are with a small enough group, you can even suggest taking a walk together. If you must stay at the table to be polite, enjoy a sugar-free mint so your taste buds know that you have finished eating.

- Focus on what you *can* do, not what you *cannot* eat. The season is about spending time with friends and family. Be grateful for what you have and for the energy, health, and new outlook on life that you are gaining.
- Plan social events to not revolve around baking and eating, but to take advantage of other opportunities: holiday shopping, volunteering, or making a scrapbook. The point is to see and talk to your friends and family, not to overeat with them.
- Be prepared for questions and comments from family members you see only once a year. Decide beforehand what, if anything, you will tell them about your surgery. Do not let any remarks throw you off, whether well-meaning but badly stated ("You look great! I sure hope this new diet lasts longer than all the others"), or clearly intended to hurt ("You took the easy way out with surgery, and you *still* look like that?").
- Keep moving, even if you only have a little bit of time. The exercise will remind you that you are still working hard to lose weight and get healthy.

Holiday Foods

The hardest part about the holidays is resisting the tempting food. You will find yourself off track if you eat like you used to. On the other hand, it is unrealistic to pass up everything. Most of us have a couple of holiday treats that we look forward to every year. We also have family meals, work functions, and parties that are obligatory.

Think of the holidays as a series of separate events rather than a season. Preparing for one event at a time and keeping to your regular routine and diet the rest of the time keeps you from slipping into a constant state of eating that lasts for all of November and December. Prepare mentally before each party or meal. Plan your strategy, whether it is sitting far from the buffet table, bringing your own food, or repeating "no, thank you" as you hold a glass of ice water and talk to the other guests during the party.

Make a game out of being picky. This is one of those times when you get to act like skinny people who seem to eat whatever they want. The truth is that they choose their treats carefully. When you see them eating pecan pie at a holiday dinner, you can be sure that they ate smaller portions at dinner and exercised more that day to make up for it. You can be like them by carefully thinking about which (if any) treats are absolutely necessary, or which are very important to you. Decide when you will have them, and how many bites of each you will have. Figure out how you will make up for the extra calories. This way, you can enjoy a bite of your aunt's Christmas pudding or your boss' Christmas fruitcake without feeling either deprived or guilty. Just remember to be picky—turn your nose up at anything that does not meet your new, high standards! And continue to avoid any foods that you cannot tolerate after surgery.

Always keep your weight loss surgery diet rules in mind. Sticking to calorie-free beverages, taking tiny portions, and eating slowly are just as effective during the holidays as they are the rest of the year. Eat your lean protein first, whether it is ham or turkey at dinner or smoked salmon or shrimp at a brunch. Allow yourself a bite or two of your favorite holiday treats only after you are sure that you have eaten enough protein.

There are better and worse choices in any situation, and your mission is to make the best possible decisions. Look for low-calorie choices and for lean proteins, along with vegetables and fruits.

No matter which foods are offered, you can always limit your portion sizes and feel free to say "No, thank you" to anyone who offers you something that is not on your diet.

Holiday foods to look for include:

- Skinless turkey, ham, fish, and roast beef
- Green salad without dressing
- Roasted or steamed vegetables
- Shrimp cocktail

Common holiday foods to avoid are:

- Goose, duck, and prime rib (more than half of their calories are from fat). Try **herb-crusted albacore** or **Southwestern shrimp** instead.
- Eggnog (350 calories, 35 g protein, 21 g fat per cup). Try our modified weight loss surgery **eggnog.**
- Pecan pie, pumpkin pie. Try a **healthy apple pie** or **pumpkin cheesecake**.
- Stuffing, dressing, gravy
- Green bean casserole. Try our low-calorie version of **green bean casserole**.
- Baked goods—cinnamon rolls and other sweet breads, fruitcake, stollen, gingerbread, and Christmas cookies
- Fudge, candy (you don't have to eat it even if someone gives it to you as a gift).
- Cranberry sauce (high-sugar)
- Excessive carbs from dinner rolls, mashed potatoes and gravy, and stuffing or dressing
- Waldorf, cream, fluff, and ambrosia fruit salads

Remember that you are in charge of yourself as you go through the holidays. You can choose your foods, eat smaller portions, and politely refuse foods that you do not want to eat. Others may pressure you to eat or make discouraging or disrespectful comments about your weight, surgery, or diet, but you do not have to listen to them. Always be polite and stick to your own plan, and you will find that the holidays get better and better after weight loss surgery.

Traveling

Vacations can be scary after weight loss surgery. At home, you are familiar with the foods and strategies that help you lose weight. Away from home, your routine is interrupted. You might not know which foods you will eat and how you will get in your exercise. In the past, vacations might have meant weight gain—but not any more.

You can lose weight while traveling, and vacations after weight loss surgery can be even more fun than they were before if you have more energy than you used to. Just stick to the same strategies that you have been using. Focus on lean proteins, fill up on vegetables, chew slowly, and keep your portions small. Also, plan ahead.

At Airports and in the Air

Does this sound familiar for a travel day? After checking in at the airport and going through security, you sit down with a frosted cinnamon roll and a large mocha. On the plane you have a glass of orange juice and a package of cookies. During your layover, you grab a slice of pepperoni pizza with breadsticks and some marinara dipping sauce. On the next flight, you munch from a large bag of trail mix with a soda. You sit down for dinner at a family restaurant on your way from the airport to the hotel, and order spinach dip with chips, ribs and coleslaw, and a glass of wine.

If that was your typical travel day before surgery, you used to take in about 4,000 calories—and get no exercise. No wonder you used to gain weight when you traveled.

But this is easy enough to fix. Follow your weight loss surgery diet rules to make this day better. Here, we suggest an alternative day of post-surgery air travel. While waiting for your first flight, have a high-protein, low-calorie breakfast, such as an egg white scramble, that you made and packed up in a disposable container the night before. On the first flight, enjoy a calorie-free beverage, such as water or decaf coffee, whenever you are offered one. Skip the airplane food. Instead, have a cheese stick and some baby carrots, which you packed the night before. When you see tempting snack foods during your layover, buy a small package of beef jerky to enjoy. On your second flight, eat a single serving of mixed nuts and an apple. On your way to the hotel, stop at a park or on a nice street and take a brisk walk before going to a restaurant for dinner. Order a Caesar salad with grilled chicken, with the dressing on the side. Once you get to your destination, you will be at 1,000 calories, including several high-protein foods.

A Weight Loss Surgery Vacation Day

A healthy vacation may sound strange or impossible, but you can have one and enjoy it, too. Just as you do during the holidays, modify your weight loss goals and expectations so that you are more likely to succeed and stay motivated. Make exercise a priority, but do not let it wreck your trip. Hit the hotel gym if you can, or focus on fun opportunities; explore the city on foot, walk on the beach, or get in some hiking, scuba diving, or kayaking.

When it comes to eating, follow the same rules as you always do. Stay hydrated, and do not drink too close to meals. Savor the delicious food, and use the tips in the restaurant section of this book to guide your choices. If you are not confident that you will be able to order a high-protein, low-calorie dish at your next meal, stop by a grocery store for some fat-free cottage cheese or yogurt, a protein bar, or a can of tuna, herring, or sardines. You can almost certainly order a salad or vegetables to eat with your protein.

If you just *have* to taste a high-calorie local specialty, satisfy yourself with a single bite. Focus instead on healthy local products to get the real flavor of the land. Look for seasonal locally-produced fruits and vegetables at farmers' markets. Open-air markets often have grilled chicken or freshly caught fish and seafood. Some vendors might sell regional nutritious specialties that you can eat, such as beef jerky, olives, or whole-grain breads. Stay away from sausages, most baked goods, and preserves; they're too high in calories and fat, starches, and/or sugars.

Figure 35 – Ideas for meals while on vacation

	Ideas
Breakfast	Full-service hotel or restaurant breakfast: egg white omelette with turkey and spinach Continental breakfast: oatmeal and hard-boiled egg whites or lean ham (or bring your own protein powder to add to the oatmeal) Grocery store breakfast: non-fat Greek yogurt and fresh fruit
Lunch	Casual restaurant lunch: salad with low-fat dressing and grilled shrimp or chicken Fast-food restaurant lunch: green salad with low-fat dressing and grilled chicken (or bring your own can of tuna). Picnic lunch: from a grocery store, local shops, or a farmers' market: grilled, skewered, or rotisserie chicken, cherry tomatoes or sugar snap peas, and a small portion of whole-grain bread.
Dinner	Casual restaurant dinner: grilled fish with steamed vegetables and black beans, sweet potatoes, or brown rice Buffet dinner: stick to green salads, lean proteins, and fresh fruit. See the restaurant section for more tips.

As a weight loss surgery patient, you have some special considerations when traveling. Timing of meals, supplements, and water is just as important as at home, but more difficult. You might want to write down a schedule or set timers to remind you when you need to eat, drink, or take supplements. Always have a source of protein available; you might want to pack a few protein bars or some powder in your suitcase.

Another consideration for weight loss surgery patients is getting sick on vacation. It often happens because you are not used to the food or water of a particular region or country. Try to avoid raw vegetables and fruits—and tap water—in countries known for high rates of traveler's diarrhea or food poisoning among tourists. Vomiting from food poisoning or overeating can stretch your stomach, pouch, or sleeve, or split surgery lines.

Weight loss surgery patients, especially vertical sleeve gastrectomy patients, need to be prepared for sudden fullness (early satiety) at any time. You might have to stop eating after just a bite of food if you suddenly feel stuffed. Roux-en-Y gastric bypass patients in particular need to be careful of dumping syndrome. Do your best to find out whether foods are high-sugar; those are most likely to cause dumping syndrome. Foods that are very sweet, fried or greasy, or starchy are risky. Lap-band patients need to avoid stringy and doughy foods that are most likely to cause obstructions or become stuck in the band.

As a lap-band patient, you should not have your band filled just before traveling because you might need a slight adjustment after a fill, and it's easier when you are at home and your regular surgeon is nearby. Also, some lap-band patients go back to a puréed foods or even a liquid diet after fills, and that is much more difficult when you are on the road. Before your trip, find out which medical center or surgeon you can visit if you need an adjustment. You may need an un-fill if you get sick or develop esophageal pain while on vacation. The section on adjustments explains more about fills and unfills with the adjustable gastric band.

Keep tracking your meals. You can use a smartphone app or an internet-based app from computers in hotels or internet cafés. An old-fashioned notebook is a failproof option if you are not sure how consistent your smartphone coverage or internet access will be. You might not be able to track your nutrients precisely if you are keeping a log by hand or are in a foreign country, but you can make good guesses. The important part is to hold yourself accountable so that you make the best possible choices each day on your trip.

Salads

Salads may be your new best friends after weight loss surgery. They can be filling, nutritious, and low in calories—the perfect recipe for weight loss and health. Be careful, though. Salads can also be high-calorie, high-fat, and even high-carb. Consider these examples and estimated calorie counts.

- ☐ Taco salad – 800 calories
- ☐ Chicken Caesar salad with dressing – 700 calories
- ☐ Cobb salad with dressing – 1,000 calories
- ☐ 1 cup mayo-based coleslaw or deli salad (potato, egg, macaroni, tuna, or chicken) – 400 to 700 calories

These steps can help you build the fresh, healthy salads you need for your diet. Start with as many salad greens as you want. They have fewer than 10 calories per cup, so you can make a big salad and still stick to your diet.

- ☐ Iceberg, red leaf, green leaf, or romaine lettuce.
- ☐ Spinach or baby spinach leaves
- ☐ Arugula or baby arugula
- ☐ Mixed greens or spring greens

Add a serving of lean protein. You know the drill!

- ☐ 2 oz. grilled chicken breast, shrimp, or fish
- ☐ ¼ cup canned tuna in water, drained
- ☐ 2 to 4 hard-boiled egg whites
- ☐ ½ cup garbanzo, kidney, black, pinto, or other beans
- ☐ ½ cup shredded fat-free cheese
- ☐ 2 oz. deli turkey, ham, or chicken breast
- ☐ 1 small veggie burger or ½ cup firm tofu

Add as many low-calorie vegetables as you like. They're high-fiber and low-calorie, and they add nutrients, texture, and flavor.

- ☐ Mushrooms, sprouts, cucumber slices, radish slices
- ☐ Cherry, grape, or diced tomatoes
- ☐ Canned artichoke hearts
- ☐ Shredded cabbage, sliced beets
- ☐ Broccoli or cauliflower florets
- ☐ Sliced bell peppers or onions
- ☐ Baby corn, bamboo shoots, or water chestnuts
- ☐ Sugar snap peas or snow peas

Add a serving of fruit (optional). It adds sweetness without many calories.

- ☐ Blueberries, strawberries, raspberries, diced apple or pear
- ☐ Navel or mandarin orange wedges

Finally, dress it up with a small serving of dressing.

- Reduced-calorie dressing, such as Italian, Ranch, or vinaigrette – or salsa
- Homemade yogurt-based dressing with fat-free plain yogurt and herbs, mustard, or part of a salad dressing mix seasoning packet.
- Soy sauce or teriyaki sauce
- Fresh raspberries smashed with a little white wine vinegar, fresh tarragon, and olive oil

Delicious combinations are practically endless. These are some suggestions.

- Green leaf lettuce with black beans, grape tomatoes, diced cucumber, green onions, chopped mango, salsa
- Romaine lettuce with chicken breast, artichoke hearts, red peppers, raspberries, and fat-free raspberry vinaigrette
- Baby bok choy with grilled shrimp, shredded cabbage, baby corn, water chestnuts, tangerine wedges, and a light dressing made with 1 tsp. soy sauce, 1 tbsp. rice wine vinegar, 1 tsp. sesame oil, garlic powder and ground ginger
- Butter leaf lettuce with turkey breast, boiled egg whites, tomatoes, mushrooms, carrots, and fat-free Italian dressing
- Baby arugula with grilled chicken, sprouts, grilled eggplant and zucchini, strawberries, and a yogurt-based dressing made with fat-free plain yogurt, Dijon mustard, lemon juice, and (optional) a packet of calorie-free sweetener

Be creative with your salads so you do not get bored, but be cautious with the ingredients that can quickly add calories to your salad. Even some of the nutritious additions can be high-calorie, high-fat, or high-carb. Some are shown below.

Figure 36 – Salad additions to use sparingly or skip

Food and Serving Size	Calories
½ cup raisins, dried cranberries, or other dried fruit	260 calories
1 tbsp. olive oil	240 calories
¼ cup peanuts, walnuts, pecans, or other nuts	160 calories
2 tbsp. regular Ranch, Italian, or French dressing	150 calories
1 oz. pepperoni, salami, or bacon	120-140 calories
1 oz. crispy noodles or croutons	120 calories
½ cup sliced avocado	120 calories
¼ cup full-fat cheddar, brie, swiss, feta, or other cheese	110 calories
¼ cup bacon bits	100 calories
¼ cup sunflower, pumpkin, or other seeds	80 calories

Salads can be very filling, so start with a small amount and eat the protein part first. Chew slowly and pause between bites, just as you always do. To make your salads bigger, add more greens and lean protein.

The serving sizes provided with these recipes are for weight loss surgery patients on the solid foods diet. You may need smaller servings, especially if your surgery was more recent. If you are sharing the dish with others, they may need larger servings.

Grilled Salmon with Dill

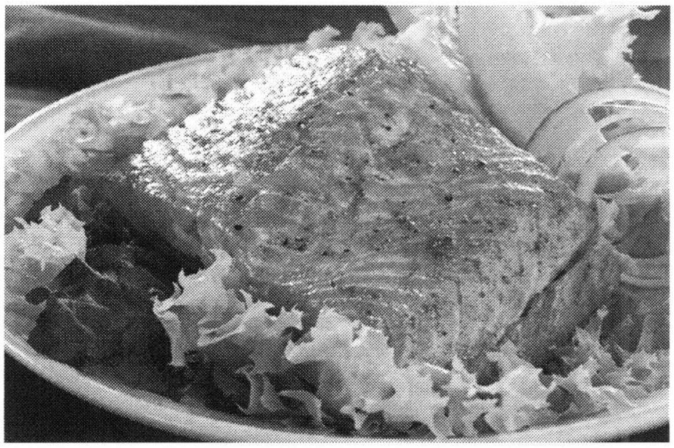

Salmon has natural heart-healthy Omega-3 fats, so you do not need to add extra fat to keep it moist when you cook it. This low-carb recipe can be made in the oven or on the grill, and it pairs well with grilled or roasted asparagus. Add a small spoonful of honey or apple juice for tasty glaze on the salmon. Orange juice adds both sweetness and citrus flavor to the glaze.
4 servings.

4 4-oz. filets of salmon
2 tbsp. Dijon mustard
¼ cup non-fat plain yogurt
¼ cup lemon juice
¼ cup chopped fresh dill, divided
Lemon wedges to garnish

Whisk the mustard, yogurt, lemon juice, and half the dill. Rinse the salmon and set it in a shallow glass dish; cover with the yogurt mixture. Cover and refrigerate for 15 minutes; turn the pieces over and refrigerate another 15 minutes.

Remove the salmon to a prepared grill pan or double sheet of foil sprayed with non-stick oil; shake off and discard excess marinade. Heat the grill and cook the salmon about 5 minutes on each side, or bake for 10 to 12 minutes in a preheated 400-degree oven. Salmon is done when it's opaque and no longer translucent, usually about 10 minutes per inch thickness of filet. Serve with lemon wedges and/or steamed asparagus.

Tuna salad

This salad is higher in protein and lower in fat than you would think based on its taste. The salad is best when made a few hours or a day before serving, so the flavors have time to blend. Have it for a snack, or serve it with a salad or with whole-wheat pretzels.

3 5-oz. cans white or light tuna in water, drained
½ cup non-fat plain Greek yogurt
2 tbsp. chopped green onion
1 stalk celery, chopped
2 tbsp. diced olives
4 hard-boiled egg whites, chopped
2 tsp. Dijon mustard
Salt and pepper to taste

Mix the ingredients together. Refrigerate before serving.

Chicken or crab salad: Instead of tuna, use 2 6-oz. cans of crab, 8 oz. imitation crab meat, or 1 12-oz. can chicken

In-a-Hurry Salad: Omit the onion, celery, and mustard. Instead, add ¼ to ½ packet of Ranch dressing mix or onion dip mix.

Stuffed cucumbers: Take a tray of these low-calorie, high-protein appetizers to a party. The host will be delighted, and you will have something healthy to eat! Mix and match the proteins and flavors to find your favorites. You can refrigerate the filling the night before and stuff the cucumbers on the day you serve them. Peel four cucumbers and cut off the ends. Cut the cucumber into three pieces of equal length, then slice each third in half lengthwise. Hollow out the cucumbers by removing the seeds with a spoon. Spread an equal portion of the protein mixture into each cucumber boat. Refrigerate until ready to serve. Makes 24.

Egg Salad

Egg salad sounds like a weight loss surgery nightmare—high-fat, high-cholesterol, and high-calorie. But it needn't be. Instead, this creamy recipe is high-protein and low-fat. Serve it on top of a bed of romaine lettuce, or scoop it up with celery or cucumber sticks.

8 eggs or 1 cup liquid egg substitute
2 tsp. Dijon or spicy brown mustard
¼ cup fat-free mayonnaise
¼ cup fat-free sour cream
1 large stalk celery, sliced
2 tbsp. diced onion
1/8 tsp. salt
1/8 tsp. black pepper

Hard-boil the eggs, peel them, and discard all but 2 yolks. Chop the eggs. (If using egg substitute, cook it with cooking spray and break it up with a fork.) Mix all the ingredients together and refrigerate for at least an hour or overnight before serving.

Greek Yogurt Dips

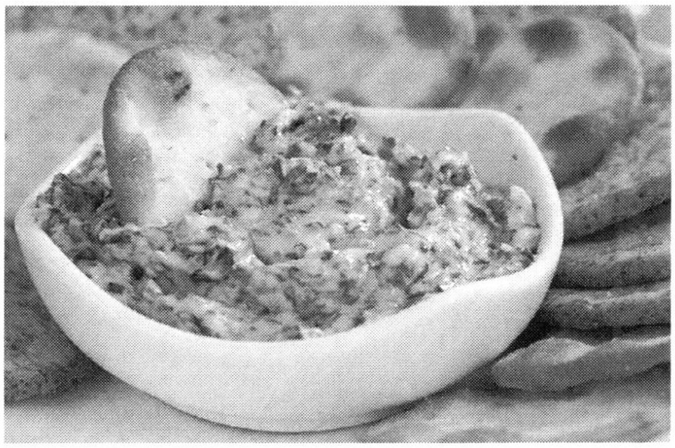

Use Greek yogurt as the base for these easy dips. For extra protein, add unflavored protein powder or skim milk powder. Serve with raw vegetables or whole-wheat crackers or pretzels. 4 servings.

2 cups non-fat plain Greek yogurt
1 packet Ranch, Italian, green onion, or onion soup dip mix

Spinach dip: Mix in 1 pkg. well-drained frozen spinach and 1 tbsp. grated carrot.

Artichoke dip: Purée and mix in 1 can artichoke hearts.

Cheesy dip: Instead of dressing mix, add ½ cup grated fat-free parmesan and 1 packet bleu cheese dressing mix.

Eggplant dip: Omit the seasoning packet, and purée the flesh of one small cooked eggplant and (optional) 1 sprig of parsley with the yogurt. Mix in 1 tbsp. olive or sesame oil, the juice of ½ lemon, ½ tsp. black pepper, and salt to taste. Great with grilled chicken skewers!

Mint cucumber dip: Omit the seasoning packet, and purée one chopped, peeled cucumber and 1 clove garlic with the yogurt. Mix in ¼ cup chopped fresh mint leaves, ¼ tsp. black pepper, and salt to taste.

Hummus dip: Drain two 15-oz. cans of garbanzo beans (chickpeas), and purée them with 1 clove garlic and the yogurt. Mix in the juice from ½ lemon and add salt to taste.

Low-Fat Bean Dip

This recipe is lower in fat than store-bought hummus. Serve it as a dip for raw vegetables, or use it as a spread on a low-carb pita stuffed with vegetables.

1 15-oz. can pinto, black, or fat-free refried beans
½ cup fat-free shredded cheddar cheese
½ cup salsa

Drain the pinto or black beans but reserve the liquid.

Purée ingredients in a food processor or with a hand blender until smooth, adding liquid if necessary. Leave some chunks if you prefer.

Deviled eggs: Hard-boil up to 12 eggs. Peel, slice in half lengthwise, and discard the yolks. Place a small spoonful of bean dip in each egg white half. See alternative deviled egg recipe next page.

Layered bean dip: Make a double recipe of bean dip and spread it in a glass baking dish. Arrange 1 cup diced tomatoes over it, with 2 cups shredded lettuce over the tomatoes. Spread 1 cup fat-free sour cream over the lettuce. Top with sliced black olives and serve with chips or crunchy raw vegetables.

Super-Skinny Deviled Eggs

Note: This recipe and photo are courtesy Juliana Walters – JuliesJazz.com – thanks Julie! This recipe would be a fine candidate for a potluck dish, or for a bring-along dish to a gathering at another place where you need to take something "safe to eat" that others will enjoy.

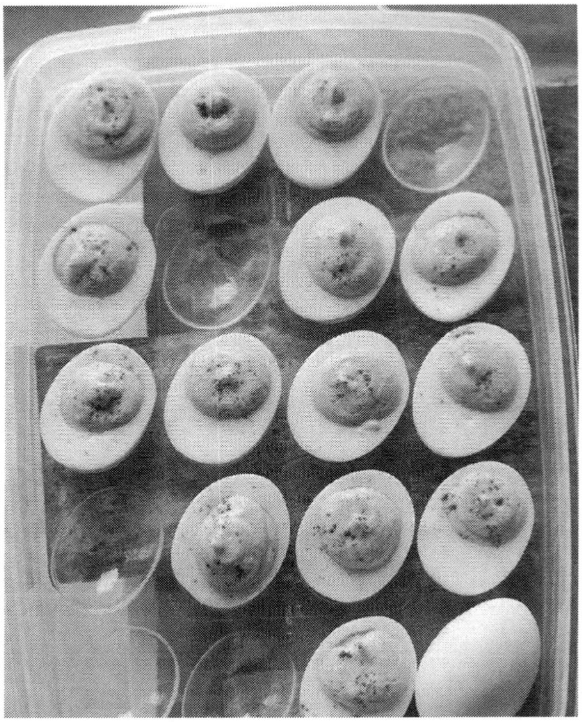

My dad challenged me awhile back to come up with a cholesterol-free, fat-free, whole foods version of deviled eggs. I think these are right on the money! The jalapeños and mustard pack the flavor punch while the Greek yogurt and garbanzos give you the rich, creamy deviled egg texture. You can eat 5 of these for around 100 calories!

12 hard-boiled eggs
½ cup garbanzo beans, drained and rinsed
3-4 tbsp. plain Greek yogurt
8 slices pickled jalapeños
2 tsp. yellow mustard
Kosher salt and black pepper to taste
Paprika (optional)

Peel the eggs and cut them in half lengthwise. Scrape out and discard all the yolks. If you mess up any whites in this process just toss them into your filling. Add the rest of the ingredients and process the entire mixture in a food processor until almost smooth. Scrape the processor mixture into a small zip-lock bag. Snip off one bottom corner of the bag with a scissors and pipe the egg whites full of filling. Sprinkle with a little paprika, if desired. Eat!!!

Pizza

This healthier version of pizza is kid-friendly, too! Save 9 grams of carbohydrates per pizza by using grilled portabella mushrooms instead of English muffins for the pizza crust. Substitute grilled chicken or ground turkey for the anchovies for a variation.

2 English muffins or 4 grilled portabellas
½ cup pizza or tomato sauce
4 oz. shredded fat-free mozzarella
½ cup diced pizza vegetables: onions, green peppers, tomatoes, spinach
2 tbsp. sliced olives, optional
1 2-oz. can anchovies, drained

Spread tomato sauce evenly over each half of English muffin. Top with cheese and then the vegetables, with optional olives and anchovies. Bake at 400 until cheese is melted. Makes four small pizzas, each with 150 calories and 13 grams of protein.

Cauliflower Crab Dip

Regular crab dip can have hundreds of calories per serving. Using cauliflower and fat-free cream cheese instead of full-fat cream cheese and mayo in this easy recipe cuts calories and fat, and increases the protein content. You can use it as a dip or instead of tuna salad on fresh lettuce or on a piece of high-fiber reduced-calorie toast. 8 servings.

1 10-oz. pkg. frozen cauliflower
8 oz. imitation crab or 2 6-oz. cans of crab meat, drained
1 2-oz. can anchovies, drained
1 3-oz. pkg. fat-free cream cheese
Black pepper to taste

Steam cauliflower until soft. Drain off excess water. Place all ingredients in a bowl and purée with a hand blender, or use a food processor until the mixture is as chunky or smooth as you like.

Lemon Rosemary Grilled Chicken

This recipe helps keep the chicken moist and tasty without adding much fat or many calories. Serve with steamed green beans or zucchini, and use the leftovers to make a chicken salad with spinach or mixed greens. You can bake this instead of grilling it. 4 servings.

1 lb. boneless skinless chicken breasts
1 tbsp. minced garlic or 4 sliced cloves
¼ cup chicken broth or stock
¼ cup lemon juice
1 tbsp. olive oil
¼ cup diced red onion
¼ cup chopped fresh rosemary
1 tbsp. Dijon mustard
1 tbsp. red pepper flakes (optional)
Black pepper and salt to taste

In a shallow glass dish, combine the garlic, chicken broth, lemon juice, olive oil, red onion, rosemary, mustard, red pepper flakes, salt, and pepper. Arrange the chicken in the dish and marinate in the refrigerator for 30 minutes. Remove the chicken and discard the marinade, then grill the chicken for 5 to 8 minutes on each side, or until no pink is visible in the center.

Mediterranean chicken skewers: Use chicken breast strips, or after removing the chicken from the marinade, cut it into smaller pieces. Wash 1 large tomato, 1 small zucchini, 1 small yellow squash, 1 onion, and 4 button mushrooms. Cut the tomato into eighths, the zucchini and yellow squash into slices, the onion into chunks, and the mushrooms into halves. Brush vegetables lightly with olive oil. Thread the chicken and vegetables onto skewers, distributing the vegetables evenly. Slide any leftover vegetables onto additional skewers. Grill the skewers for 10 to 15 minutes, turning frequently, or bake at 400 until done.

Meatloaf

High-protein? Check. Vegetables? Check. Guilt-free comfort food? Check. Family friendly? Check. It's even pre-portioned if you make it in muffin tins. Serve it with puréed cauliflower and sliced cooked carrots. Freeze leftovers in individual bags and save for another dinner or for a snack or lunch with a salad. 12 servings.

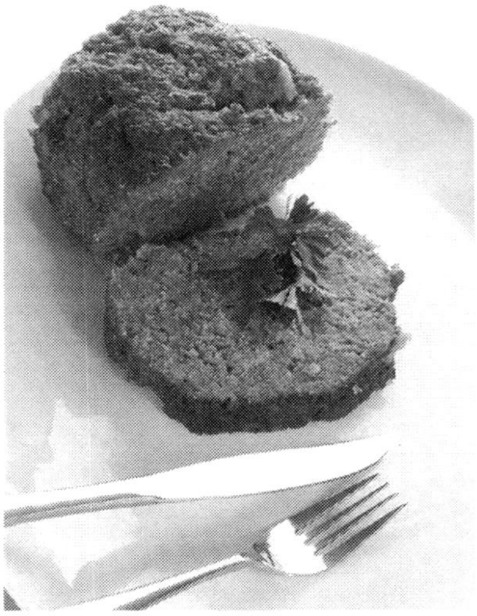

1 lb. lean ground turkey or soy crumbles
1 cup Fiber One or other high-fiber cereal, crushed
2 egg whites or 1/4 cup liquid egg substitute
1 medium zucchini, peeled and grated
1 onion, chopped
1 8-oz. can tomato sauce
1 tsp. Italian seasoning
1/2 tsp. salt

Beat the egg whites or egg substitute; mix all ingredients in a bowl. Spray a muffin tin with non-stick cooking spray. Divide the mixture evenly into muffin cups and bake at 375 until the meatloaf is thoroughly cooked, about 30 minutes.

Kale Chips

Don't hit the potato chips! Satisfy your crunchy cravings with these low-calorie, high-fiber alternatives. Try different seasonings to keep them interesting. Serve with grilled chicken for a low-calorie dinner, or pair with fat-free cottage cheese for a high-protein snack. 4 servings.

1 bunch kale or 1 bag of washed pre-cut kale leaves
2 tsp. olive oil
1 tsp. sea salt or seasoned salt
Optional: black pepper and/or garlic powder to taste

If you are using a bunch of kale, wash the leaves and dry them. Remove and discard the stems and tear the leaves into bite-sized pieces. In a bowl, toss the leaves with the olive oil until evenly coated, then add seasoning and toss lightly. Bake on a cookie sheet with fat-free non-stick spray at 350 for 10 to 12 minutes or until crispy.

Variations: substitute one of these seasonings for the salt: 1 tbsp. low-sodium soy sauce, 2 tbsp. light Italian dressing, 2 tbsp. low-fat shredded parmesan, 1 tbsp. balsamic vinegar.

Basic Stir-Fry

This is a flexible recipe that you can modify depending on what you have on hand. You can make it easier by starting with cooked leftover chicken, shrimp, or fish and a frozen bag of stir-fry vegetable mix. Serve with ¼ cup cooked brown rice. 4 servings.

16 oz. raw chicken, shrimp, or white fish, or 12 oz. cooked chicken, shrimp, or fish
2 diced green onions
2 tsp. sesame or olive oil
2 tbsp. soy sauce
½ tsp. ground ginger
½ tsp. garlic powder
1 cup Napa cabbage, green cabbage, or bok choy, cut into pieces
2 cups vegetables in pieces: broccoli florets, sliced mushrooms, or sugar snap peas

Heat the oil in a wok or large skillet. If using raw chicken, shrimp, or fish, cook in the pan over medium heat, stirring regularly until cooked. Remove from pan. Add the vegetables to the pan. Stir regularly until they begin to soften, about 5 minutes. Add soy sauce, ginger, and garlic, continuing to cook and stir until the vegetables are lightly cooked. Add the chicken, shrimp, or fish to the pan and stir to mix well. Serve when all ingredients are hot.

Baked Cabbage, Cauliflower, or Broccoli

There's something compelling about baking an entire head of cabbage, cauliflower, or broccoli. This recipe is easy and delicious. Serve it with cod, trout, or almost any other lean protein. 6 servings.

1 large head cauliflower, 1 medium head cabbage, or 1 large bunch broccoli (about 2 lbs.)
1 tbsp. olive oil
1 cup beef broth
1 tsp. seasoned salt or Italian seasoning, or ½ tsp. each of salt and black pepper

Rinse the vegetables. Trim the cauliflower, remove the outer leaves from the cabbage, or remove the fibrous stalks from the broccoli. Cut the cauliflower or cabbage in half or quarters for faster cooking. Set the vegetable in a baking dish; brush it with olive oil and sprinkle the seasoning over it. Pour the beef broth around the edges. Bake at 400 for 40 to 60 minutes, or until done, basting regularly with the broth during baking.

Oven-Fried Chicken Tenders

Traditional fried chicken is high-fat and high-calorie. It can cause dumping syndrome and, if you have the gastric band, cause a blockage. Turn instead to this recipe to feed your craving. Serve it with puréed cauliflower, baked sweet potato fries, or coleslaw made with fat-free mayo or a light Italian dressing. 4 to 6 servings.

1 lb. boneless skinless chicken breast strips
2 egg whites or ¼ cup liquid egg substitute
2 tbsp. milk
1 cup crushed high-fiber cereal, such as Fiber One, or bread crumbs made from reduced-calorie high-fiber bread
1 tsp. onion powder
1 tsp. Italian seasoning
¼ tsp. salt
¼ tsp. pepper, optional

Spray a baking sheet with non-stick fat-free spray. Blend the cereal, onion powder, salt, and pepper in a shallow bowl. Set aside. Briefly beat the egg whites and milk together in a small bowl. Add the chicken breast pieces to the bowl and mix until all chicken pieces are coated with egg wash. One at a time, dip the chicken pieces into the bowl with the dry ingredients. Turn them until they are coated all over, then arrange them on the pan. Bake at 375 about 30 minutes, or until fully cooked.

Smashed Cauliflower

A large portion of mashed potatoes can have over 500 calories and more than half the carbohydrates you need in a day. Instead, serve up a portion of smashed cauliflower. It is a high-fiber, low-calorie dish to satisfy your craving for mashed potatoes. Serve this smashed cauliflower with lean beef or a chicken breast, or use it in recipes instead of mashed potatoes, as in our shepherd's pie or cottage pie recipe. Stick to low-sodium canned gravy or even beef broth instead of traditional high-fat gravy. 6 servings.

1 medium head cauliflower, washed and cut into florets, or 1 16-oz. bag of fresh cauliflower
2 tbsp. reduced-fat buttery spread, melted
¼ cup chicken broth
½ tsp. salt
1 tsp. Dijon mustard
Optional: diced chives for topping

Steam the cauliflower, with other vegetables if you are using them (see below), until tender. Drain excess water. While the cauliflower is still hot, stir in cheese and reduced-fat butter spread. Add chicken broth and salt. Use a potato masher or gently blend the mixture to thick and chunky consistency. If desired, sprinkle chives on top before serving.

Cheesy smashed cauliflower: Stir in 2 wheels of light Laughing Cow Mini Babybel cheese, your choice of flavors, at room temperature, when you add the buttery spread.

Smashed cauliflower with parsnip, turnip, sweet potato, or carrots: Cook 1 parsnip, 1 turnip, 1 sweet potato, or 2 carrots, peeled and in chunks, with the cauliflower.

Healthy Apple Pie

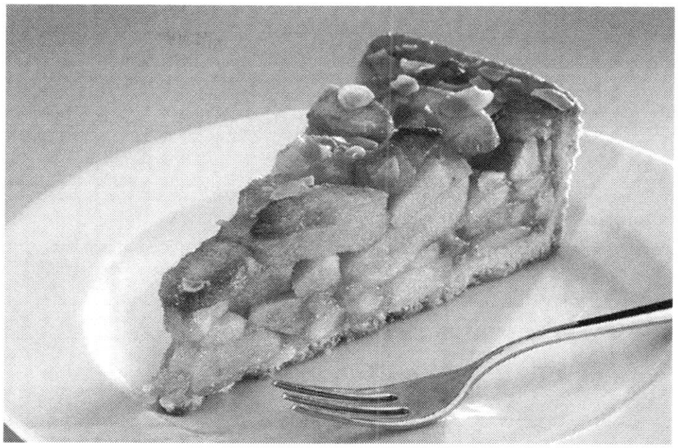

Traditional apple pie recipes use tart apples and a lot of sugar, but this recipe uses sweet apples. It will be sweet enough with the cinnamon and the optional low-calorie sweetener. You can save more calories by making this recipe without the crust. Have the stewed apples as a low-calorie dessert, add them to plain non-fat yogurt or fat-free cottage cheese for a high-protein breakfast or snack, or pair them with pork tenderloin for a festive dinner. You can also purée them in a food processor for a delicious applesauce. 8 servings.

Crust:
1 cup Fiber One or other high-fiber cereal
½ cup rolled oats
Optional: 2 packets of low-calorie sweetener
¼ cup fat-free milk
2 tbsp. reduced-fat buttery spread

Spray an 8-inch pie pan with non-stick cooking spray. Use your hands to combine the ingredients in a bowl until uniformly mixed. Press the crust evenly into the pan, pushing it up slightly around the edges of the pan, and bake at 375 for 10 minutes.

Apples:
6 medium Gala, Fuji, or other sweet variety apples
¾ cup water
2 tsp. ground cinnamon
¼ cup (6 packets) low-calorie sugar substitute
½ tsp. vanilla extract

Core the apples. Lap-band patients and patients just starting the solid foods diet should peel the apples. Slice thinly. Heat the water in a pot. Add the other ingredients. Cook over medium heat, stirring frequently, until apples are tender, about 12-15 minutes. Spoon the apple filling into the prepared crust. Optional: top with chopped almonds. Bake at 375 for 20 minutes.

Note: you can also layer the apples in a pattern over the pie crust and sprinkle the other ingredients over the top before baking.

Only the Good Stuff Lasagna

This high-protein, high-fiber version of lasagna is comforting without loading you with all the fat, carbohydrates, and guilt of regular lasagna. The recipes cuts calories by swapping eggplant for lasagna noodles and extra lean ground turkey for regular ground beef. Use meatless soy crumbles to make this dish vegetarian. This is a meal in itself. 12 servings.

2 large eggplants
2 egg whites
1 tbsp. water
½ cup crumbs from reduced-calorie bread
1 tsp. Italian seasoning
1 onion, diced
2 cloves garlic, crushed
1 tbsp. olive oil
16 oz. extra lean ground turkey or meatless crumbles
½ tsp. black pepper
1 tsp. dried basil
1 28-oz. can low-fat meatless tomato sauce
1 15-oz. can diced Italian-style tomatoes
8 oz. white or cremini mushrooms, sliced
½ cup shredded fat-free mozzarella
¼ cup grated fat-free parmesan

To prepare the eggplant: slice it into ¼-inch thick pieces. Mix bread crumbs and Italian seasoning. In a separate bowl, lightly beat egg whites and water. Dip the eggplant slices in the mixture, then dip them into the crumbs to coat them. Set the eggplant aside.

Heat the oil in a pan. Add onion and crushed garlic and cook, stirring often, until onions are transparent. Add the turkey or soy crumbles, pepper, and basil, and cook until meat is browned. Stir in half the tomato sauce. Combine remaining tomato sauce with the tomatoes and mushrooms.

Spray a 9-inch square baking pan with non-stick cooking spray. Spread half the meat mixture at the bottom, then layer half the eggplant slices over that and the mozzarella over that. Spread half the tomato mixture next, then layer the remainder of the meat mixture over that. Then arrange the remaining eggplant slices and tomato sauce. Add parmesan on top, then bake at 375 for 30 minutes or till heated and bubbly.

Cheesy Spinach Mushroom Caps

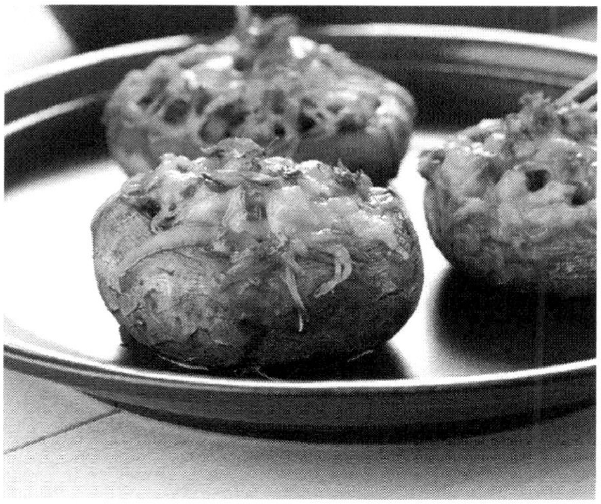

With so much focus on protein after weight loss surgery, you might find yourself getting tired of meat. That's why we're including this vegetarian version of stuffed shells with a white sauce instead of tomato sauce. The fat-free ricotta provides plenty of protein, and using portabella mushrooms instead of pasta shells saves calories and fat; the small ones are often called cremini mushrooms. If you have any leftover filling, bake it on the side and use it as a sandwich filling, salad topping, or a dip for vegetables. 6 servings.

6 large or 12 small portabella mushrooms
1 15-oz. container fat-free ricotta
1 cup fat-free cottage cheese
2 egg whites
½ tsp. garlic powder
1 tsp. onion powder
2 tbsp. chopped fresh basil
¼ cup fat-free milk
8 oz. fresh spinach leaves, washed
¼ cup breadcrumbs from reduced-calorie toasted bread
¼ cup fat-free parmesan
1 tsp. Italian seasoning
2 Roma tomatoes
1 28-oz. can spaghetti sauce, optional

Wash the portabellas—or use a vegetable brush to clean them—and remove the stems. Set aside.

Lightly beat eggs and milk together. Add cheeses and onion, garlic and basil, and mix until blended and smooth. Stir in spinach leaves. Finely chop the tomatoes, drain, and stir in. Spoon cheese mixture into each portabella cap to fill it. Place the caps in a baking dish that has been sprayed with non-fat spray. (If using spaghetti sauce, put it on the stove over low heat).

Mix together breadcrumbs, cheese, and Italian seasoning and distribute the mixture evenly over the top of each portabella cap. Bake at 350 for 25 minutes or until mushrooms are tender. Serve with the spaghetti sauce if desired.

Spaghetti Squash Recipes

Who says you can't have anything good after weight loss surgery? If pasta was your ultimate comfort food in the past, spaghetti squash is the perfect substitute. When you cook it and scoop out the flesh, you get yellow strands that you can use like spaghetti. Unlike spaghetti, which is 180 calories and 35 grams of carbohydrates per cup, cooked spaghetti squash is just 42 calories and 10 grams of carbohydrates per cup. Make the basic recipe and serve it as a side dish, or try one of the following high-protein nutritious dishes.

Basic Spaghetti Squash
4 servings

1 large spaghetti squash
Non-stick, fat-free cooking spray
Salt and pepper, optional

Spray a baking sheet with cooking spray. Cut the spaghetti squash in half lengthwise and set the halves, cut side down, on the baking sheet. Bake at 375 for 40 minutes. Turn the squash halves over, spray the tops with non-stick cooking spray, add the salt and pepper if desired, and bake for another 10 minutes or until tender.

Remove from the oven and let cool at least 5 minutes. Scoop out the flesh with a fork to serve or use in a recipe. You can also just fluff up the squash insides with a fork and serve as is.

Spaghetti Squash and Cheese
4 servings

1 recipe basic spaghetti squash, above
4 wedges of Laughing Cow Light bleu cheese
½ cup fat-free cream cheese
½ cup fat-free cheddar, shredded
½ cup fat-free milk
½ cup chicken broth
Optional mix-in: 2 cups fresh spinach leaves
Optional topping: ¼ cup crushed Fiber One mixed with ½ tsp. onion powder and 2 tbsp. fat-free parmesan cheese

Mix the cheeses, milk, and broth in a bowl. Microwave for 30 to 60 seconds, or until cheeses are gently melted. Stir until blended. Add the optional spinach leaves to the cheese mixture, then add the mixture to the spaghetti squash flesh. Toss to combine, then arrange the mixture in a sprayed 9-inch baking dish. Cover with topping, if desired. Bake at 375 for 20 minutes or until bubbly. Serve with fresh tomatoes or a small green salad.

Skinny Spaghetti Squash and Meatballs
4-6 servings

1 recipe basic spaghetti squash, above
1 lb. extra lean ground turkey or soy crumbles
1 10-oz. can tomato soup
1 pkg. onion soup mix
¼ cup crushed Fiber One or other high-fiber cereal
1 tsp. Italian seasoning
½ tsp. oregano
½ tsp. garlic powder
2 egg whites
1 28-oz. can or jar of low-fat spaghetti sauce

Lightly beat the egg whites. Dissolve the onion soup mix in the tomato soup. Add the mixture to the soy crumbles or turkey and mix thoroughly. Add the remaining ingredients, except the spaghetti sauce, and mix. Form into 12 meatballs and arrange on a sprayed baking dish; cover with the spaghetti sauce. Cover loosely with foil, and bake at 375 for 25 minutes or until done. To serve, spoon sauce and 1 or 2 meatballs over each portion of spaghetti squash.

Sweet Spaghetti Casserole
This makes a good and simple breakfast, snack, or dessert. Try it with apples or strawberries, or add some oats. 4-6 servings.

1 recipe basic spaghetti squash, above
1 lb. fat-free cottage cheese
½ cup milk
1 tsp. cinnamon
½ tsp. pumpkin pie spice
Low-calorie sweetener to taste, or about ¼ cup (6 packets) granulated sweetener.

Mix the cheese, milk, spices, and sweetener together. Stir it with the spaghetti squash, then bake in a sprayed 9-inch loaf pan at 350 for 20 minutes.

Broccoli Avocado and Egg Toast

NOTE: This recipe and photo courtesy of Juliana Walters – JuliesJazz.com – thanks Julie!

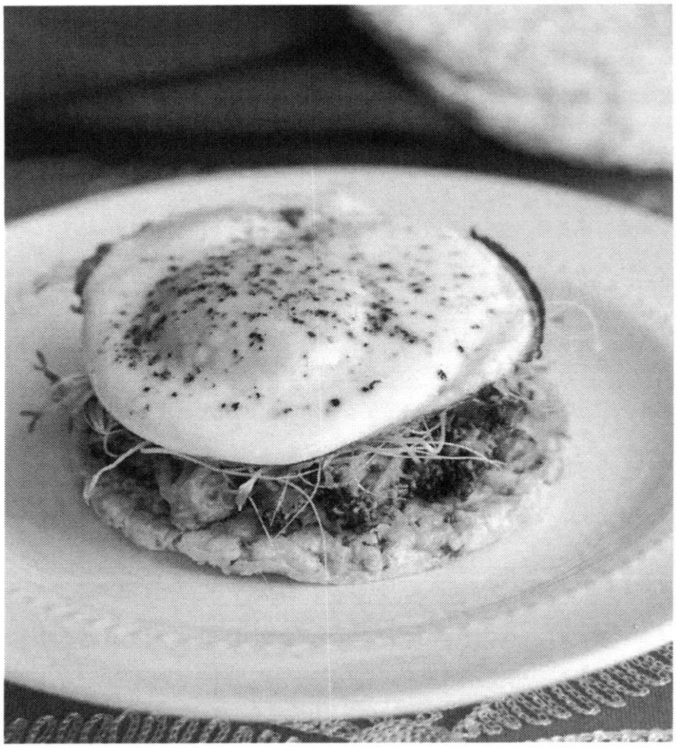

When I'm in serious diet mode I love to eat rice and corn cakes. I know they aren't super-nutritious, but you can pile on the yummy lean ingredients you would typically put on bread—like broccoli, avocado, and egg—but you don't get all the extra empty calories of the bread. They are my go-to bread substitute. A poached egg is best, but you can also "fry" it in a sprayed pan, add 1 tbsp. water, cover with a lid, and "steam" the egg.

6 oz. broccoli florets (roasted)
1 oz. mashed avocado
2 eggs (steamed or poached)
2 rice cakes or corn thins
Kosher salt and pepper
Alfalfa sprouts (optional)

Preheat oven to 450 arrange the raw broccoli on a small parchment-lined cookie sheet sprinkled with salt and pepper. Roast for 20 to 25 minutes until the broccoli is tender and the ends are browned.

In a medium mixing bowl, stir together the mashed avocado and broccoli. Divide broccoli and avocado mixture in half and spread each half onto your cakes. Top the cakes with a little handful of sprouts and the eggs. EAT!!!

Southwestern Shrimp

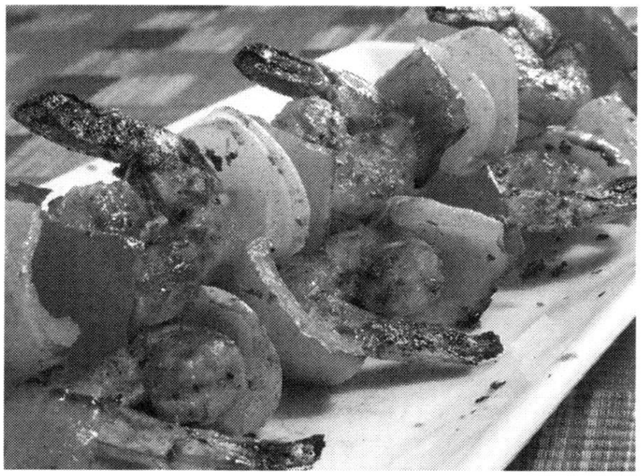

The lime and cilantro give these shrimp a nice Southwestern flavor. Serve them with black beans, salsa, and grilled zucchini and yellow squash, or skewer the shrimp with chunks of green and red and yellow peppers—or add some onion and pineapple for variety! Other variations are suggested below. Do not overcook the shrimp; they need to be just opaque before serving. This makes 4 servings.

1 tbsp. olive oil
2 cloves garlic, peeled and sliced
1 lb. peeled raw shrimp
3 chipotle peppers, canned in adobo sauce and diced
2 tbsp. lime juice
1 tsp. paprika
½ cup chopped fresh cilantro, divided
½ tsp. black pepper
½ tsp. red pepper flakes (optional)

Heat olive oil in a large skillet over medium heat. Add garlic and cook, stirring occasionally, until translucent. Add the shrimp, peppers, paprika, half the cilantro, black pepper, and red pepper flakes. Cook over medium heat, stirring occasionally, until shrimp are just barely cooked. Add lime juice and cilantro, and cook for another 30 seconds before serving.

Shrimp Fajitas: Before starting the Southwestern shrimp, peel and slice one onion and cut 1 red bell pepper and 1 green bell pepper into strips. Add the onions when you add the garlic to the pan, cooking a little longer till onions are barely translucent. Add the bell peppers and lime juice when you add the shrimp. Serve on its own or with a small, low-carb, high-fiber tortilla.

WLS-Style Rolled Shrimp Tacos: Remove 8 large whole leaves from a head of iceberg lettuce. Prepare 1 cup diced tomatoes, 2 tbsp. sliced black olives, ¼ cup fat-free cheddar cheese, and 2 tbsp. diced green onions. Arrange one-fourth of the shrimp and a small amount of the other ingredients in each of four lettuce leaves; add a small spoonful of plain Greek yogurt to each. Roll up each leaf, then roll up a second leaf around the first to help keep it closed. Serve with salsa and extra Greek yogurt.

Shrimp Salad: Put 1 lb. chopped romaine into a large salad bowl. In another bowl, mix ½ cup black beans, ½ cup yellow corn, and 1 chopped mango. Spoon the bean mixture over the romaine lettuce and toss briefly. Arrange the cooked shrimp over the salad just before serving with a low-fat vinaigrette on the side.

Roasted Vegetables

You can use almost any vegetables in this recipe: bell peppers, zucchini, tomatoes, sliced red onions, yellow squash, eggplant, button or portabella mushrooms, asparagus spears (not lap-band patients), onions, Brussels sprouts or string beans, carrots, potatoes, yams, or sweet potatoes. If you choose potatoes, yams, or sweet potatoes, count them as a starch instead of a vegetable. These are excellent if they're roasted in the oven, and even tastier if grilled outdoors. (Note baking times at end of recipe.) 4 servings.

1 lb. fresh vegetables
2 tbsp. olive oil
2 cloves garlic, crushed
¼ cup chicken broth or bouillon
¼ cup balsamic vinegar
2 tbsp. minced fresh rosemary
1 tsp. dried thyme (or 1 tbsp. fresh)
½ tsp. black pepper

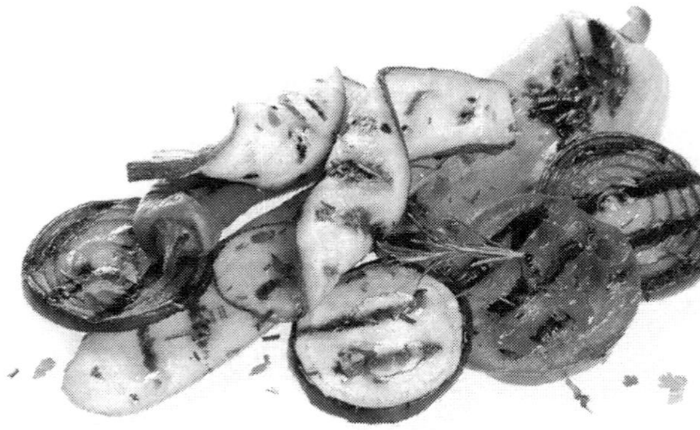

Wash and prepare vegetables as necessary; i.e., peel the carrots and onion, trim the asparagus tips, trim beans, cut off the tips of the mushroom stems and Brussels sprouts, and discard the ends of the zucchini and yellow squash. Set aside.

Mix remaining ingredients together in a large bowl. Add vegetables and toss until evenly coated. Arrange in a roasting pan and cover loosely with foil. Bake at 400 for 20 minutes; remove foil and bake another 10 minutes. Potatoes and sweet potatoes may need additional cooking time; if you are including these it's a good idea to start them first, bake 10 minutes, then add the other vegetables. Asparagus and tomatoes need less baking time and it's advisable to add them separately for the last 10 minutes of roasting.

Grilled Italian Summer Squash

Eggplant, zucchini, and yellow summer squash are abundant and delicious during grilling season. Enjoy slices of these veggies with ground turkey patties while everyone else is chowing down on hamburger buns with fatty ground beef burgers. You can also make this recipe in the oven, roasting at 400 for 20 minutes or until tender. 8 servings.

2 lbs. eggplant, zucchini, or summer squash combination (e.g. one of each)
½ cup fat-free Italian dressing

Wash the vegetables and discard the ends. Slice them into ¼-inch thick rounds, toss with dressing, and grill for 4 minutes on each side or until golden and tender.

WLS Chili

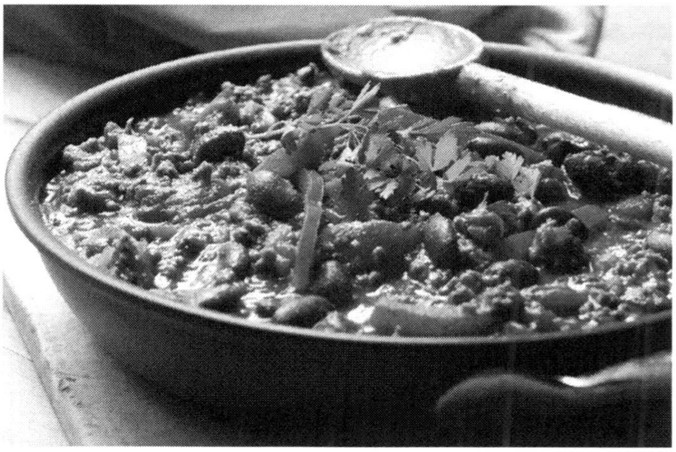

This chili is just as filling, warming, and comforting as regular chili, but it is low-fat and high-fiber. It is a one-dish meal in itself with the protein, vegetables, and starch from the beans. It tastes even better the next day, so make a big batch and enjoy it two days in a row, or freeze the extra for another meal. Once you've put it together, you can simmer it in the oven or a crockpot for a couple hours to blend flavors.
16 servings.

1 onion, diced
3 cloves garlic, peeled and crushed
1 tbsp. olive oil
16 oz. extra lean ground turkey or vegetarian soy crumbles
1 green bell pepper, seeded and chopped
1 red bell pepper, seeded and chopped
2 stalks celery, sliced thinly
1 jalapeño pepper, seeded, veined, and diced (optional)
1 15-oz. can black beans, drained and rinsed
1 15-oz. can garbanzo beans, drained
1 15-oz. can kidney beans, drained
1 cup beef broth, divided
3 15-oz. cans plain or Mexican-style stewed or diced tomatoes
2 tbsp. chili powder
½ tsp. cayenne
1 tsp. cumin
2 bay leaves

Heat oil in a large, heavy-bottomed pot. Add onion and garlic and cook over medium-high heat, stirring often, until onions are translucent. Add ground turkey, peppers, celery, and ¼ cup beef broth. Cook, stirring often, until turkey is browned. Add remaining ingredients. Bring to a boil, then simmer, stirring occasionally, for at least 90 minutes. Garnish with fresh cilantro and tomatoes or thin-sliced red peppers.

Protein Oatmeal Pancakes

Oatmeal pancakes are hearty and delicious, and very nutritious with the addition of egg whites and protein powder Serve them fresh for a weekend brunch, or make them the night before to enjoy in the morning. They travel well, so you can take them to work for a mid-morning snack. Place a slice of fat-free cheese on one for a creative sandwich, or spread with low-fat peanut butter and a few blueberries. 8 small pancakes.

½ cup rolled oats
½ cup fat-free milk
¼ cup sugar-free protein powder: vanilla, banana, or chocolate
4 egg whites or ½ cup liquid egg substitute, mixed
½ tsp. baking powder
½ tsp. salt
1 or 2 packets low-calorie sweetener

In a bowl, add the oats to the milk and let stand. Mix together protein powder, baking powder, salt, and sweetener. Whisk the egg whites till foamy and then whisk in the mixed dry ingredients. Combine ingredients and mix lightly; the batter should be medium-thin. Add more milk if batter is too thick.

Heat a large skillet sprayed with fat-free spray. Add two spoonfuls of batter to the pan for the first two pancakes. Cook until each pancake is bubbly in the middle and beginning to dry around the edges; flip the pancakes and cook until done. Remove from the pan and repeat for the remaining pancakes. Serve immediately with fruit or yogurt, or let cool and then refrigerate in zip bags or waxed paper.

Cottage Cheese Pancakes

This recipe provides protein from cottage cheese, egg whites, and protein powder—and satisfies your morning sweet tooth. Add fruit or serve with fruit, and have a slice of turkey bacon on the side for a delicious breakfast. 8 small pancakes.

1 cup fat-free cottage cheese
4 egg whites or ¼ cup liquid egg substitute
½ cup milk
1 tsp. vanilla
½ cup whole-wheat flour
½ tsp. salt
½ tsp. baking powder
2 tbsp. sweetener
½ cup fruit (optional) diced apple or pear, blueberries, or chopped ripe peach

Beat cottage cheese, egg whites, milk, and vanilla together in a bowl. Blend the dry ingredients together and add to the liquid mixture. Blend well.

Heat a skillet sprayed with fat-free spray. Add two spoonfuls of batter to the pan for the first two pancakes. Cook until each pancake is bubbly in the middle and beginning to dry on the edges, then flip the pancakes and cook until done. Remove from the pan, and repeat with the remaining batter. Serve immediately, or cool and refrigerate to store.

Zucchini Pancakes

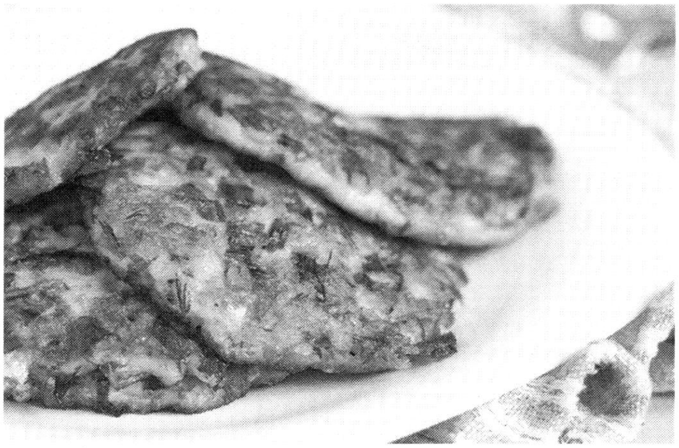

This recipe can help you get your veggies in if you are having trouble because you do not like them or you cannot think of tasty ways to fix them. Cooked spaghetti squash can substitute for the zucchini. Try these for a light snack, for breakfast or lunch with cottage cheese or tuna, or for dinner as a side dish with chicken. You can add shredded carrots to this, or minced red bell peppers, or a little shredded (imitation or real) crab.

4 servings.

1 cup grated zucchini
1 cup chopped fresh spinach leaves
1/4 cup grated onion
2 egg whites
1/4 cup cooked barley or 1/4 cup dry rolled oats
1/2 tsp. salt
1/2 tsp. baking powder
1/2 tsp. dried oregano
1/2 tsp. dried thyme
1/4 tsp. ground nutmeg

Beat egg whites till foamy. Mix in the remaining ingredients and blend. Heat a skillet sprayed with fat-free spray. Add two large spoonfuls of batter to the pan for the first two pancakes. Cook until each pancake is bubbly in the middle and beginning to dry around the edges; flip the pancakes and cook until done. Remove from the pan, and repeat with the remaining batter.

Protein Powder Muffins

Have one of these muffins instead of something from a bakery or coffee shop, and you'll save hundreds of calories at breakfast. Spread fat-free cream cheese on it and serve it hot with scrambled egg whites on the side, or pack one to enjoy for a mid-morning snack with low-fat string cheese. 12 muffins.

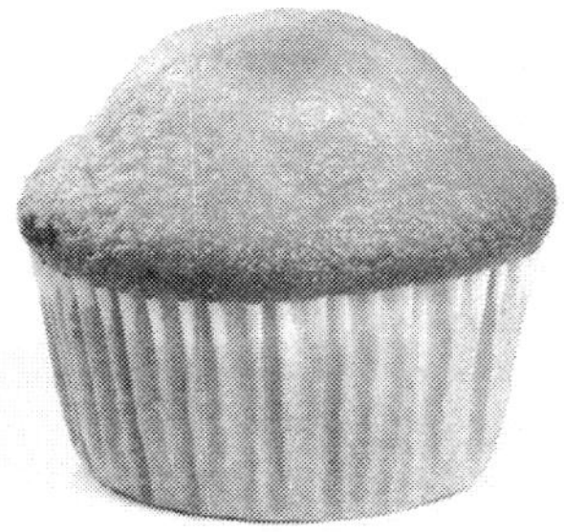

½ cup rolled oats
½ cup warm milk
2 egg whites
1 egg
½ tsp. vanilla
½ cup whole wheat flour
2 tsp. baking powder
½ tsp. salt
¼ to ⅓ cup sugar substitute or 6-8 packets of sweetener
3 tbsp. sugar-free vanilla protein powder

Add the oats to the milk and let stand for 10 minutes. Mix flour, baking powder, salt, sugar substitute, and protein powder together. In a separate bowl, combine the egg whites, egg, and vanilla; mix thoroughly. Combine the dry ingredients, wet ingredients, and oatmeal, and stir till blended.

Spoon the batter into muffin tins sprayed with non-stick spray. Each muffin cup should be no more than 2/3 full. Bake at 375 for 20 minutes or until a toothpick inserted in the center comes out clean.

Banana muffins: Use banana-flavored sugar-free protein powder; mash a small ripe banana and add that to mixture when combining all ingredients.

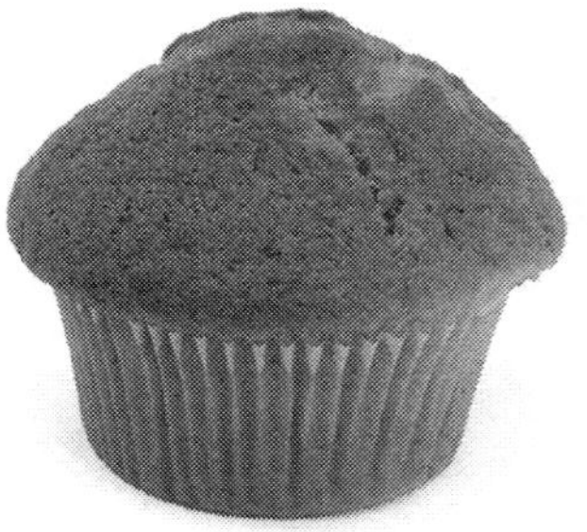

Chocolate muffins: Use chocolate-flavored sugar-free protein powder, and mix ¼ cup unsweetened baking cocoa and an extra sweetener packet into the dry ingredients.

Spiced muffins: Add 1 tsp. cinnamon, ½ tsp. ginger, ½ tsp. nutmeg, and a pinch of cloves to the dry ingredients; use ½ cup canned pumpkin purée or ½ cup applesauce instead of the egg whites.

Note on oats: Rolled oats (old-fashioned or quick) add soluble fiber, which forms a gel in the digestive tract. Soluble fiber helps block absorption of cholesterol, and the Mayo Clinic recommends a daily minimum of 10 grams of soluble fiber for cholesterol-reducing benefits. Rolled oats and quick oats are approximately equivalent in nutritional value, but rolled oats add more texture and interest to food items. Both are equally digestible.

Green Bean Casserole

Digging into a traditional version of this casserole can break your diet, but this reduced-calorie version for a holiday dinner gives you something guilt-free to eat with your turkey or ham. This is a big recipe, so there is plenty to pass around; leftovers are delicious. 8 servings.

2 slices low-calorie bread
4 tbsp. cup light buttery spread, divided
2 tbsp. diced green onion
2 tbsp. minced fresh thyme
½ cup chicken or mushroom broth
1 small onion, peeled and diced
8 oz. sliced mushrooms
4 oz. fat-free cream cheese
1 tsp. onion powder
½ tsp. garlic powder
1 tbsp. soy sauce
1 cup fat-free milk
½ cup fat-free plain Greek yogurt or sour cream
24 oz. fresh or frozen green beans
½ cup diced lean ham (optional)
¼ cup fat-free shredded mozzarella

Toast the bread and crumble the toast into a small bowl. Add 1 tbsp. buttery spread and the green onion and thyme, and mix until uniform. Some chunks are okay.

Heat the broth in a pot. Add the onion and mushroom, and simmer until cooked. Add the cream cheese, onion and garlic powders, soy sauce, milk, and yogurt or sour cream. Heat until cream cheese is melted. Add the green beans (and ham if using); and cook over medium heat until beans begin to soften.

Pour the mixture into a sprayed casserole dish and sprinkle the crumbly toast mixture on top. Cover with mozzarella. Bake at 375 for 25 minutes or until bubbling hot.

Pumpkin Cheesecake

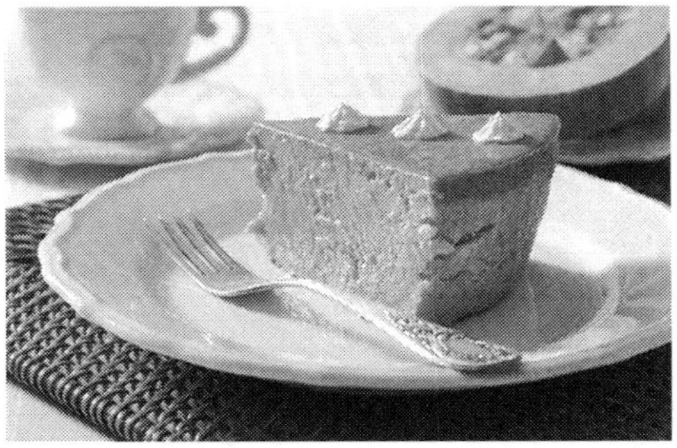

This is a great one for holidays, since a slice of this instead of regular pumpkin pie can save hundreds of calories and a lot of sugar. It's also healthy enough to enjoy at any time. Try it without the crust to save a few calories, or try it with puréed sweet potatoes or winter squash for a different flavor. Danish or acorn squash makes a delicious pie! You can use low-fat cream cheese or ricotta and make it without the crust for a delicious low-fat (and nutritious) dessert. 6 servings.

Crust:
1 cup Fiber One or other high-fiber cereal
2 graham crackers
Optional: 2 packets of low-calorie sweetener
¼ cup fat-free milk
2 tbsp. reduced-fat buttery spread

Spray an 8-inch pie pan with non-stick cooking spray. Use your hands or a pastry blender to combine the ingredients in a bowl until they are uniformly mixed. Press the crust evenly into the pan and bake at 375 for 10 minutes.

Filling:
1 15-oz. can pumpkin purée (or 1¾ cups sweet potato or squash purée)
4 egg whites or ½ cup liquid egg substitute
½ cup milk
½ cup fat-free ricotta or cottage cheese
1 tsp. cinnamon
1 tsp. pumpkin pie spice
¼ tsp. salt
2 scoops sugar-free vanilla protein powder
½ cup sugar substitute, or 12 packets of sweetener

Beat the first four ingredients until smooth. In another bowl, combine the spices, salt, protein powder, and sweetener and mix into the pumpkin mixture. Pour the batter into the pie shell. Bake at 325 for 50 minutes or until the pie is just barely set. Do not overbake.

Note: you can substitute fat-free sugar-free non-dairy creamer for the milk. Hazelnut or pecan flavor is excellent!

Mini Cheesecakes

Sometimes you need a creamy treat with easy-to-store leftovers and no guilt. These single-serving mini cheesecakes are perfect for those times. 12 servings.

½ pkg. sugar-free instant vanilla pudding mix
½ cup fat-free milk
8-oz. cream cheese
1 lb. (2 cups) non-fat cottage cheese
½ cup low-calorie sweetener (12 packets)
½ tsp. vanilla extract

Beat the pudding mix into the milk. Then beat all of the ingredients together until smooth. Distribute the batter evenly into a sprayed or papered 12-cup muffin tin. Refrigerate for 30 minutes or until set.

Triple chocolate cheesecakes: use sugar-free chocolate pudding mix instead of vanilla and add 4 tbsp. (¼ cup) unsweetened cocoa powder when you blend the ingredients. After pouring the batter into the muffin tin, drizzle with a blended mixture of 2 tbsp. baking cocoa, 1 tbsp. milk, and 2 to 3 low-calorie sweetener packets (or 2 tbsp. granulated low-calorie sweetener).

Spicy pumpkin cheesecakes: Cut the milk to ¼ cup and add ½ cup pumpkin, 1 tsp. cinnamon, and ½ tsp. pumpkin pie spice.

Note on vanilla: Real vanilla extract is more expensive because it's a labor-intensive process to create it from vanilla beans or pods, which take a long time to grow on the plants. Imitation vanilla is cheaper, tastes slightly bitter, and is produced from coal tar.

Baked Tuna Casserole

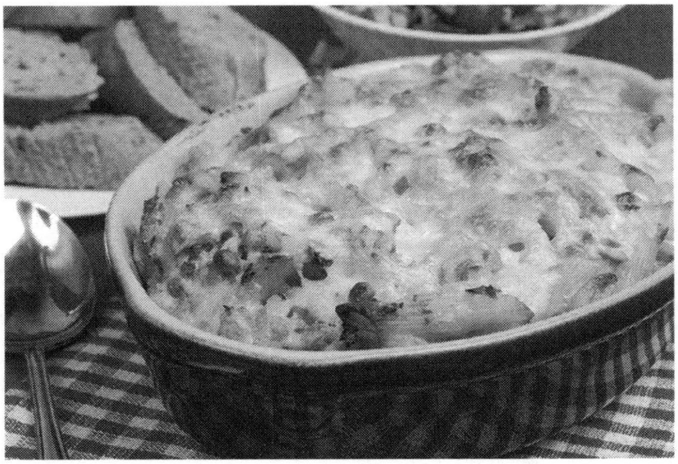

This recipe also works well with canned salmon or mackerel instead of tuna. The barley, whole-wheat pasta, or oats provide good texture. For the topping, choose between a creamy cheddar cheese and a pecan crust. Feel free to mix in 1 to 2 cups vegetables, such as peas, broccoli, spinach leaves, or canned artichoke hearts, when you stir in the soup. 8 servings.

2 5-oz. cans white or light tuna in water, drained
½ cup chicken or vegetable stock
1 small onion, peeled and diced
2 stalks celery, diced
8 oz. sliced mushrooms
1 10-oz. can condensed low-fat cream of mushroom soup
½ cup cooked barley, 1 cup cooked whole-grain pasta, or ½ cup dry oats
½ cup fat-free shredded cheddar or ⅓ cup crushed pecans

In a stockpot, heat the chicken or vegetable stock. Add onion and celery and cook over medium heat for 10 minutes. Add the mushrooms, cream cheese, and soup; cook and stir until the cream cheese is soft and melting. Add tuna and the barley, pasta, or oats.

Transfer to a 9-inch square baking dish sprayed with non-stick spray. Sprinkle the cheddar or crushed pecans on top. Bake at 375 for 20 minutes or until bubbly and golden on top.

Four-Bean Salad

Bean salad is a high-fiber, high-protein choice that can be a snack on its own or part of a meal served with fruit, cottage cheese, or tuna. This version saves you calories by using sugar substitute instead of sugar, and by cutting back on the oil. Make it the night before to let the flavors blend overnight in the refrigerator. 8 servings.

½ white onion, peeled and thinly sliced
1 15-oz. can garbanzo beans, drained
1 15-oz. can kidney beans, drained
1 15-oz. can cut yellow wax beans, drained
1 15-oz. can cut green beans, drained
½ cup white vinegar
2 tbsp. olive oil
3-4 packets sugar substitute
½ tsp. each salt and black pepper

Mix the ingredients together in a bowl. Refrigerate for at least two hours before serving.

Mediterranean Bean Salad: Cut the sweetener in half, and add the juice of ½ lemon plus 2 tbsp. minced fresh parsley, 2 tbsp. minced fresh oregano, and ½ cup fat-free feta cheese.

Mexican Bean Salad: Cut sweetener in half; add 1 can drained corn, 1 Roma tomato, chopped, ¼ cup minced fresh cilantro, ½ tsp. cumin, the juice of 1 lime, and ½ tsp. garlic powder.

Scrambled Eggs

This recipe makes one breakfast serving. You can double it if you are cooking for two or if you want leftovers. Try eating the warm eggs with turkey breakfast sausage and strawberries, or make a portable wrap with the leftovers and some spinach. This recipe is quite versatile; make it plain, use some of our suggested variations, or come up with your own ideas. 1 serving.

4 egg whites
2 tbsp. fat-free milk
Pinch of salt
¼ tsp. black pepper

Whisk the ingredients together in a bowl. Spray a non-stick pan with cooking spray and warm it over medium-low heat. Pour the eggs into the pan and cook, folding the eggs over nearly constantly, until eggs are just set. For variations, mix one or more of the following into the egg mixture after whisking or during cooking:

Protein options: 1 oz. cubed ham; 1 oz. cooked, diced chicken breast; 1 oz. smoked salmon; ¼ cup cooked lean ground turkey

Cheesy treats: 1 wedge any flavor Laughing Cow light cheese; ½ oz. low-fat shredded cheddar or mozzarella; 2 tbsp. low-fat parmesan

Veggie combos: 1 cup fresh spinach leaves; ½ cup cooked broccoli; ½ cup mixed vegetables; ½ cup diced tomatoes and bell peppers; ½ cup cooked zucchini

Herbs: Freshly chopped cilantro, parsley, basil, oregano, thyme, or dill; use a sprinkle of dried herbs or 1 tbsp. fresh herbs.

Tofu Scramble

This recipe is a high-protein alternative to eggs or meat for breakfast. Pack up the leftovers for lunch on a salad or fold into a high-fiber, low-carb wrap. 4 servings.

1 tbsp. sesame, olive, or canola oil
1 clove garlic, pressed or minced
½ onion, chopped
4 oz. mushrooms, sliced
1 block firm tofu, drained well and patted dry
1 tsp. soy sauce
½ tsp. onion powder
½ cup chopped red pepper or 1 cup fresh chopped spinach leaves

Heat the oil in a large skillet. Add onion, mushrooms, and garlic; cook until translucent. Add tofu and soy sauce, onion powder, and red pepper or spinach. Cook, breaking up the tofu, until spinach is wilted or red pepper is tender. Serve warm.

Protein Powder Shakes

You will probably be drinking protein shakes during the liquid phase of the post-op diet before you transition to solid foods. You might continue to depend on shakes for extra protein if you are a vertical sleeve gastrectomy patient who fills up quickly or a lap-band patient who just got a fill, or if you just need a little extra protein. Keep it interesting with these variations! 1 serving each.

Basic vanilla shake:
1 scoop sugar-free protein powder
¾ cup fat-free milk
1-2 packets artificial sweetener

Blend all ingredients in a blender.

Chocolate Shake: Use chocolate protein powder, and add 2 tbsp. unsweetened cocoa powder.

Mocha Shake: Add 1 heaping tsp. instant coffee granules to the chocolate shake.

Extra Creamy Shake: Cut the milk to ¼ cup and add a 5-6 oz. fat-free yogurt and ¼ pkg. sugar-free instant pudding mix.

Pumpkin Pie Shake: Add ¼ cup pumpkin purée with ½ tsp. cinnamon, ¼ tsp. nutmeg, and a dash of cloves.

Favorite Fruit Shake: Add ¼ pkg. strawberry sugar-free instant pudding mix plus 4 strawberries. Substitute your favorite fruit!

Piña Colada Shake: Cut milk to ¼ cup and add fat-free piña colada yogurt and ¼ pkg. sugar-free vanilla instant pudding mix.

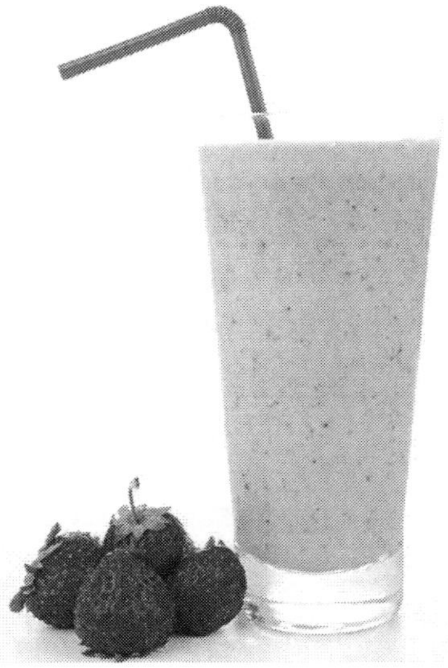

Protein Fruit Smoothies

With plenty of protein and fruit, these smoothies are substantial enough for breakfast or other meals. Mix and match the fruit and yogurt flavors to make fun combinations. Be sure to use pasteurized eggs or liquid egg substitute, not unpasteurized raw eggs. 1 serving.

Basic Smoothie:
5-6 oz. fat-free yogurt
¼ cup liquid egg substitute
1-2 packets artificial sweetener
1 cup fresh or frozen fruit
2 tbsp. ground flaxseed (optional)
2 to 4 ice cubes

Blend all ingredients in a blender and serve.

Suggested flavor combinations:
Blueberry yogurt with frozen blueberries
Berry yogurt with ½ banana and ½ cup frozen mixed berries
Lime yogurt with frozen strawberries
Strawberry yogurt with fresh or frozen mango
Vanilla yogurt with fresh or frozen peaches
Strawberry yogurt with fresh or frozen melon

Eggnog

A single cup of eggnog can have 400 calories! You don't want to have to skip this holiday treat, so why not make your own version? This recipe has about 120 calories per cup. Be sure to use pasteurized eggs or liquid egg substitute, not unpasteurized raw eggs. 4 servings.

4 cups fat-free milk
1 cup liquid egg substitute
4 scoops sugar-free vanilla protein powder
1 pkg. sugar-free vanilla instant pudding mix
2 tbsp. rum
2 tbsp. sugar-free rum-flavored syrup
½ tsp. nutmeg
¼ tsp. cinnamon

Blend ingredients well until light and creamy. Serve immediately or chill for later.

Protein French Toast

Order a French toast breakfast in a restaurant, and you can get over 1000 calories and 50 grams of fat. Serve this recipe with some fruit and a strip of turkey bacon, and you will have a high-fiber, high-protein breakfast with a fraction of the calories. If you don't have stale bread, just leave it uncovered on the counter overnight. 4 servings.

4 slices stale reduced-calorie bread
1 scoop vanilla protein powder
4 egg whites or ½ cup liquid egg substitute
¼ cup fat-free milk
¼ cup sugar-free breakfast syrup
¼ cup artificial sweetener or 6 packets, divided
½ tsp. cinnamon

Beat the protein powder, egg whites, milk, syrup, and half of the sweetener lightly together in a bowl. In a separate small bowl, combine the remainder of the sweetener and the cinnamon.

Spray a skillet with non-stick cooking spray and warm it over medium heat. Dip the bread into the egg mixture. Turn to coat both sides of each slice. Set one or two slices of the battered bread in the skillet and cook over medium heat until the bottom sides are golden brown. Flip and brown the other sides. Remove from the pan, spray it again if necessary, and cook the other slices of bread. Serve warm with fruit or cottage cheese.

Baked Oatmeal Bars

Make these ahead of time for an on-the-go breakfast or snack. Serve with fat-free cream cheese and strawberries, or spread a bit of peanut butter on one for some healthy fats and extra protein. The "brown sugar" artificial sweetener adds extra flavor, and you can stir in nuts and raisins if your diet will tolerate them. 8 servings.

2 cups fat-free milk
4 egg whites or ½ cup liquid egg substitute
½ cup applesauce
1½ cups rolled oats
1 cup Fiber One or other high-fiber cereal
3 scoops sugar-free protein powder
¼ to ½ cup (6-12 packets) artificial sweetener
½ tsp. baking powder
½ tsp. salt
½ tsp. cinnamon
¼ tsp. nutmeg
1 banana, thinly sliced (optional)

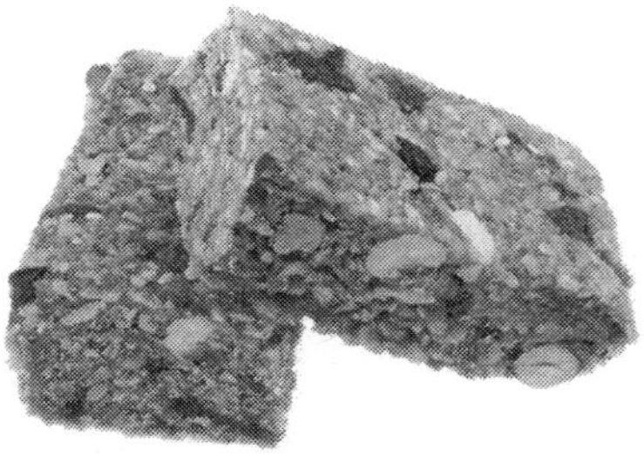

Mix the dry ingredients together. Set aside. Beat egg whites or liquid eggs; mix in the milk and applesauce. Add dry ingredients. Add banana, if desired. Spray an 8-inch square cake pan with non-stick cooking spray. Spread the batter in the pan, and bake at 375 for 20 to 25 minutes or until done.

Herb-Crusted Albacore

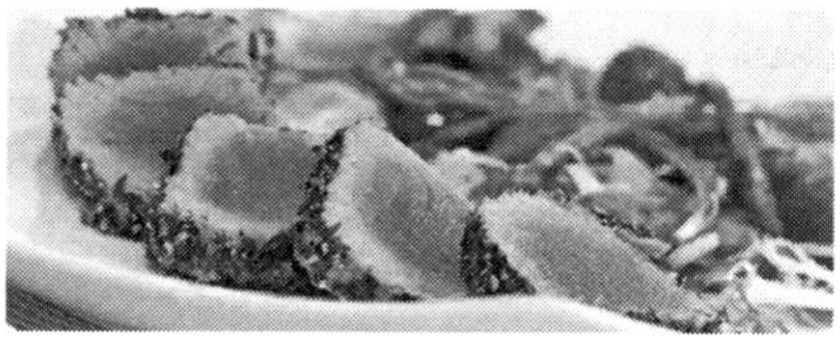

2 small albacore medallions
4 tsp. chopped basil
4 tsp. chopped parsley
2 tsp. chopped oregano
2 tsp. minced garlic
1 tbs. olive oil
Salt and pepper to taste

Mix basil, parsley, oregano, garlic, and olive oil together. Coat outside of albacore with herb mixture; season to taste with salt and pepper. Spray a skillet with non-stick spray and heat over medium-high to high heat; add tuna with the herb side down and sear for 90 seconds. Reduce heat to medium, turn the albacore over and sear the other side until cooked to just medium rare.

If available, buy albacore in whole loins. With the frozen loin about half thawed, use the herb coating on the outside, and slice into 1-inch medallions. Albacore loins are far easier to slice if they're still about half frozen.

Chocolate Fudge Treat

This recipe can satisfy your chocolate craving while providing protein with not much fat or sugar. Increase cocoa slightly and/or add 1 tsp. instant coffee to add deeper chocolate taste. This treat is thick and gooey; serve warm on its own or with ½ banana or some strawberries.

4 servings.

1 pkg. instant sugar-free chocolate pudding mix
2½ cups fat-free milk
2 egg whites
½ cup fat-free sour cream
½ tsp. vanilla
½ cup (12 packets) sugar substitute
3 scoops sugar-free chocolate protein powder
¼ cup unsweetened baking cocoa
½ cup flour
½ tsp. each salt and baking powder

Mix dry ingredients in a bowl. Set aside. Beat pudding mix with milk for 1 to 2 minutes. Beat in eggs, then mix in sour cream and vanilla. Add dry ingredients and mix gently. Spray an 8-inch pan with non-stick spray. Pour batter into pan and bake at 350 for 20 minutes or until thickened.

Food Lists

These food lists show the nutritious foods that should make up most of your low-calorie, high-protein, nutritionally balanced weight loss surgery diet.

Lean Proteins

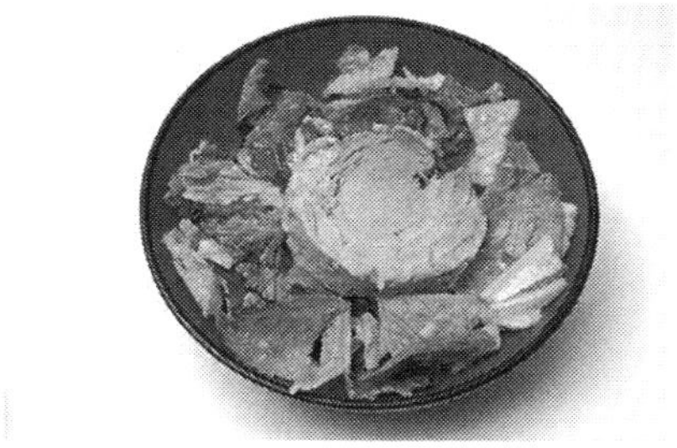

Protein helps stave off hunger while it nourishes you. Aim for 1 to 2 servings at most meals and snacks, for 4 to 7 servings daily. Eat your protein foods first at each meal and snack, so you are sure to get them in even if you fill up quickly and cannot finish your entire meal. Each of these choices is nearly pure protein. A serving has about 7 grams of protein, almost no fat, and about 30 to 45 calories.

- ☐ 1 oz. lean meat, such as lean sirloin or tenderloin
- ☐ 1 oz. skinless chicken or turkey breast
- ☐ 1 oz. extra lean ground beef, chicken, or turkey
- ☐ 1 oz. fish or shellfish
- ☐ 2 egg whites or ¼ cup fat-free, cholesterol-free liquid egg substitute
- ☐ 1 oz. canned flake meat or low-fat seafood such as chicken, tuna, or crab
- ☐ 1 oz. canned herring, salmon, mackerel, sardines, or anchovies (contain some fat, but rich in heart-healthy omega-3 fats)
- ☐ 1 oz. deli turkey breast or lean ham

Medium-High Sources of Protein

These foods help you meet your protein requirements, but they are lower in protein per serving than the pure protein options above. Other healthy nutrients in these foods include dietary fiber or heart-healthy fats.

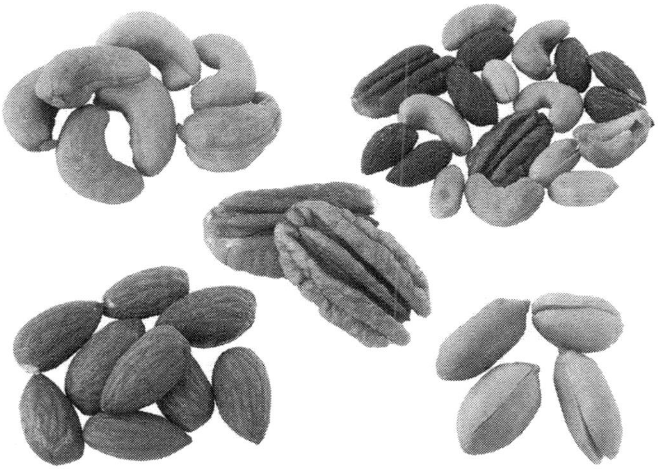

- ☐ 1 tbsp. peanut butter
- ☐ 4-6 almonds, cashews or pecans, or 2 tbsp. peanuts, walnuts or other nuts
- ☐ 2 oz. or ¼ cup soft or firm silken tofu
- ☐ ¼ cup cooked beans or lentils
- ☐ ¼ cup hummus or garbanzo bean dip
- ☐ 1 oz. soy-based meat substitute: meatless soy crumbles, vegetarian chicken, and veggie burgers

Dairy

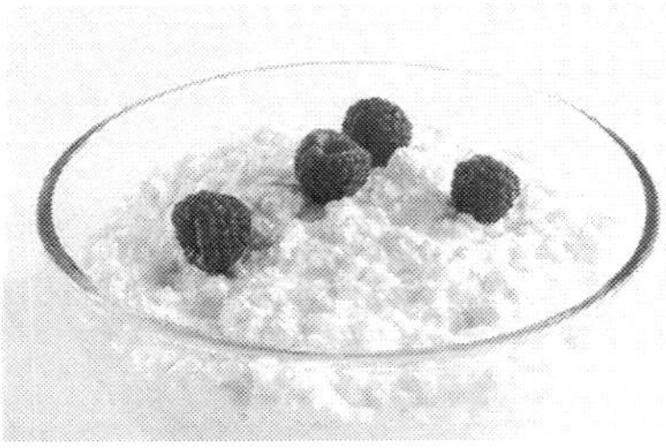

Reduced-fat dairy products are high in protein and calcium. Choose only milk on your liquid diet, and avoid sugar-sweetened yogurt. Aim for 2 to 4 dairy servings per day for strong bones.

- ☐ 1/4 cup fat-free cottage cheese or ricotta cheese
- ☐ 1 oz. low-fat or fat-free cheese or 1/4 cup shredded cheese
- ☐ 1/2 cup fat-free plain or no sugar-added flavored regular or Greek yogurt
- ☐ 1 cup fat-free milk or calcium-fortified soy or almond milk

Vegetables

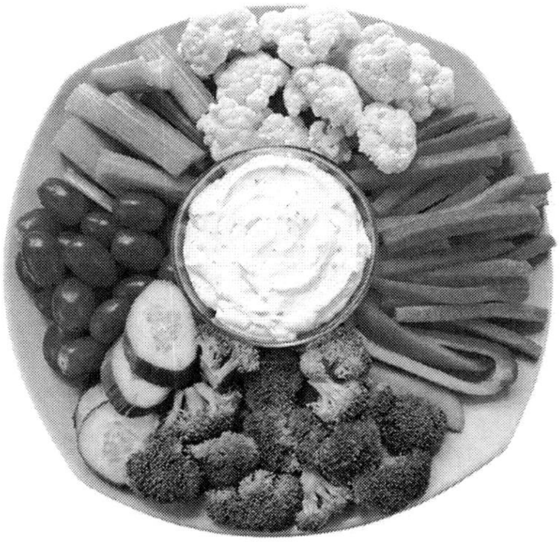

Non-starchy vegetables are low in calories and high in fiber and other nutrients such as vitamins, minerals, and antioxidants.

Because they are so low in calories, they are excellent for weight loss. If you are still hungry, you can always take a second helping of vegetables.

Vegetable juices are best when you are on the liquid phase of the post-surgery diet; later you can choose fresh vegetables.

Frozen vegetables are next, and canned vegetables are also good choices.

Try to get in 1 to 2 servings at more than half of your meals and snacks, and eat your vegetables right after you eat your protein.

- ☐ 1 cup raw or 1/2 cup cooked or canned: carrots, green beans, broccoli, cauliflower, zucchini, snow peas, string beans, onions, artichokes, mushrooms, eggplant and turnips, asparagus, celery, cucumbers, bell peppers, sprouts, jicama, kale, cabbage, spinach, beets, or radishes
- ☐ 2 cups salad greens: red or green leaf lettuce, romaine, arugula, endive, watercress
- ☐ 1/4 cup tomato sauce or salsa
- ☐ 6 oz. (3/4 cup) tomato or vegetable juice

Fruits

Fruits are sweet enough to be low-calorie substitutes for desserts and sweet snacks. After the liquid diet stage, choose fresh fruit or unsweetened canned fruit. Fruit juices and dried fruit are nutritious, but they are high in calories and sugar. Aim for 2 or 3 servings per day.

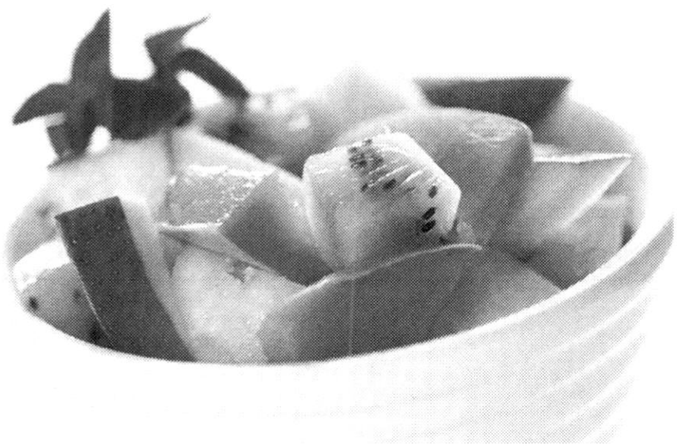

- ☐ 1 small apple, orange, nectarine, peach, kiwi, or pear
- ☐ 2 apricots, plums, tangerines, or figs
- ☐ 1/2 banana, mango, or grapefruit
- ☐ 1/2 cup applesauce, canned fruit cocktail or peaches or cherries
- ☐ 3/4 cup blueberries, raspberries, blackberries, pineapple, or grapes
- ☐ 1 cup cantaloupe, watermelon, honeydew, or strawberries
- ☐ 2 tbsp. raisins or other dried fruit
- ☐ 4 oz. (1/2 cup) fruit juice

Starches

Starches are higher in calories and carbohydrates, but they provide essential nutrients and energy. Colorful starchy vegetables and fortified whole grains are the most nutritious starches. White bread, white rice, white pasta, refined cereals, and white potatoes are considered less nutritious—but they do provide soluble fiber, so don't eliminate them entirely. Get 2 to 5 servings per day, and measure your portions carefully!

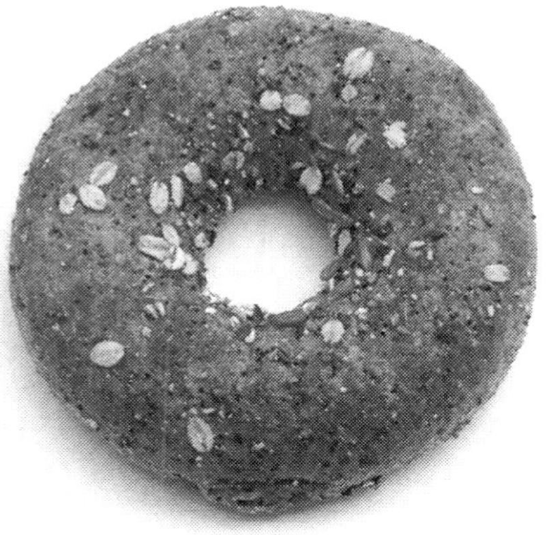

- ☐ 1/2 slice regular (not reduced-calorie) bread or toast
- ☐ 1 slice low-calorie bread or toast
- ☐ 1/2 English muffin
- ☐ 1/4 bagel
- ☐ 1/2 cup cooked hot cereal (oatmeal, cream of wheat, farina)
- ☐ 3/4 cup unsweetened cold breakfast cereal
- ☐ 1/3 cup cooked pasta, bulgur, wheat bran, barley, quinoa, white or brown rice
- ☐ 1/2 cup sweet potato or white potatoes
- ☐ 1 cup cooked acorn or butternut squash
- ☐ 3/4 oz. hard pretzels
- ☐ 1/2 cup puffed cereal, or 1/4 cup bran cereal or granola
- ☐ 4 crackers (saltines, Ritz crackers or graham cracker quarters)
- ☐ 3 cups air-popped popcorn
- ☐ 1/2 cup canned or cooked corn

Fats

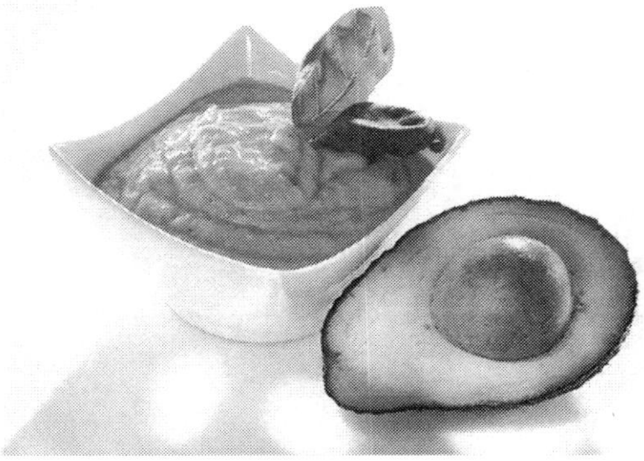

Fats are high in calories, but you need them for proper nutrient absorption. Limit fats that are solid at room temperature, e.g. butter and margarine. Instead, choose plant-based oils and other fat sources. Aim for 2 to 3 servings each day, and keep in mind that a serving of fats is small.

- ☐ 1 tsp. (⅓ tbsp.) oil (olive, canola, corn, sesame, peanut, sunflower)
- ☐ 1 tsp. trans-fat-free margarine
- ☐ 1 tbsp. low-fat mayonnaise or salad dressing
- ☐ 2 tbsp. mashed avocado or guacamole
- ☐ 1 tsp. butter (high in saturated fat)
- ☐ 1 tbsp. cream cheese
- ☐ 2 tbsp. sour cream
- ☐ 1 tbsp. flaxseed (or pumpkin, sesame, or sunflower seeds)
- ☐ 1 tbsp. tahini (sesame seed paste)

Conclusions

Weight loss surgery is a major event, and it is far more than a single event. Deciding on which type of weight loss surgery, choosing a surgeon, preparing for your surgery, and undergoing the operation are monumental, but they are only the beginning. From recovering from surgery to losing the extra pounds to keeping them off, weight loss surgery is a part of your life forever.

The path to losing weight and keeping it off can be challenging at times, but the rewards can be worth the investment many times over. We have written this book to make the journey easier. The small pieces of encouragement, ideas for maintaining better relationships with yourself and others, and tricks for enjoying vacations, holidays, and the other fun parts of life without breaking stride in your quest for a healthy lifestyle are all intended to help you take a long-term view and live life to its fullest. Food, of course, is a daily challenge, and the recipes, meal plans, and food tips in this book can help you keep your diet exciting without feeling deprived.

If you enjoyed this book, we suggest looking at a copy of our other books:

- *The Big Book on the Lap-Band: Everything You Need to Know to Lose Weight and Live Well with the Adjustable Gastric Band*
- *The Big Book on the Gastric Sleeve: Everything You Need to Know to Lose Weight and Live Well with the Vertical Sleeve Gastrectomy*
- *The Big Book on the Gastric Bypass: Everything You Need to Know to Lose Weight and Live Well with the Roux-en-Y Gastric Bypass*

We also invite you to visit **BariatricPal.com**, a vibrant community with members, like you, who are considering weight loss surgery or who have already had it. At BariatricPal, you are sure to meet new friends and learn many more tips and tricks for living the good life after weight loss surgery!

Best of luck in your journey.

Sincerely,

Alex Brecher and Natalie Stein

About the Authors

Alex Brecher

The founder and CEO of BariatricPal, the world's largest online social network dedicated to the weight loss surgery community, Alex Brecher became committed to fighting obesity with weight loss surgery after his own successful lap-band surgery. It helped him to lose over 100 pounds and keep it off for over 10 years.

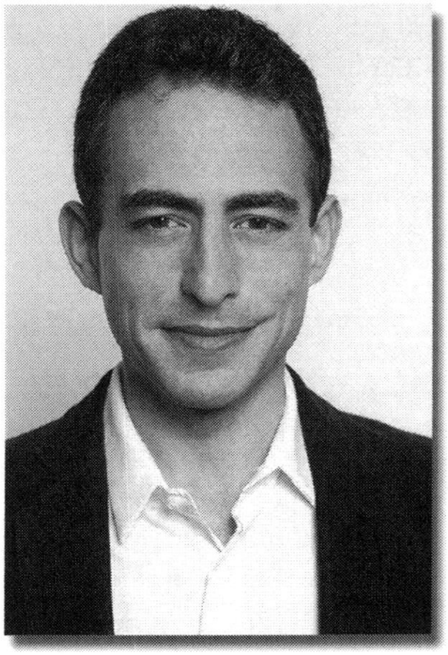

Brecher's years of experience in web design, forum hosting, technology, and management enabled him to establish BariatricPal and guide its development. Brecher has served as a consultant for numerous bariatrics companies, and he supports many professional organizations for weight loss surgery, including the American Society for Bariatric and Metabolic Surgery (ASMBS), International Federation for the Surgery of Obesity and Metabolic Disorders (IFSO), and the Association for the Study of Obesity (ASO).

Brecher is a native New Yorker who loves spending time with his three children and staying fit by working out at the gym and running. Brecher and Stein have co-authored three previous books on weight loss surgery.

Natalie Stein

Natalie Stein is a writer who specializes in nutrition and weight loss. For years, she has worked with co-author Alex Brecher to maintain the content on BariatricPal and its predecessor, WLSBoards. Stein received graduate degrees in nutrition and public health, and teaches graduate courses in public health nutrition at a major university. In addition to co-authoring three books on weight loss surgery with Brecher, Stein has a college textbook on public health nutrition to her credit.

Stein is based in Los Angeles. She enjoys talking to friends and family and spending time at the gym, and she is an avid runner who has completed six marathons.

54443760R00082

Made in the USA
Middletown, DE
04 December 2017